Slowing Down to Run Faster

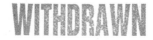

Slowing Down to Run Faster

A SENSE-ABLE APPROACH TO MOVEMENT

Edward Yu

North Atlantic Books
Berkeley, California

Somatic Resources
San Diego, California

Published by

North Atlantic Books   and   Somatic Resources
Berkeley, California   San Diego, California

Cover photo © gettyimages.com/Halfpoint
Cover design by Nicole Hayward
Book design by Happenstance Type-O-Rama

Interior photos by Andreia de Abreu Gomes and Edward Yu

Models: Raquel Brito, Andreia de Abreu Gomes, and Edward Yu

Author photo by Ricardo Jesus

Sketch of Rodin's *Pierre Wiessant* by Andreia de Abreu Gomes

Feldenkrais®, Feldenkrais Method®, Functional Integration®, Awareness Through Movement®, and Guild Certified Feldenkrais Practitioner® are service marks of the FELDENKRAIS GUILD® of North America.

Printed in Canada

Slowing Down to Run Faster: A Sense-able Approach to Movement is sponsored and published by the Society for the Study of Native Arts and Sciences (dba North Atlantic Books), an educational nonprofit based in Berkeley, California, that collaborates with partners to develop cross-cultural perspectives, nurture holistic views of art, science, the humanities, and healing, and seed personal and global transformation by publishing work on the relationship of body, spirit, and nature.

North Atlantic Books' publications are available through most bookstores. For further information, visit our website at www.northatlanticbooks.com or call 800-733-3000.

MEDICAL DISCLAIMER: The following information is intended for general information purposes only. Individuals should always see their health care provider before administering any suggestions made in this book. Any application of the material set forth in the following pages is at the reader's discretion and is his or her sole responsibility.

Names: Yu, Edward, 1967- author.
Title: Slowing down to run faster : a sense-able approach to movement / Edward Yu.
Description: Berkeley, California : North Atlantic Books, [2020] | Includes bibliographical references and index. | Summary: "To run faster, better, and more efficiently, you have to learn to run faster, better, and more efficiently. Trainer and former triathlete Edward Yu shows you how to achieve the results you want with a new multidisciplinary approach"— Provided by publisher.
Identifiers: LCCN 2019050970 (print) | LCCN 2019050971 (ebook) | ISBN 9781623174903 (trade paperback) | ISBN 9781623174910 (ebook)
Subjects: LCSH: Running—Training. | Running speed. | Running—Physiological aspects.
Classification: LCC GV1061.5 .Y8 2020 (print) | LCC GV1061.5 (ebook) | DDC 796.42—dc23
LC record available at https://lccn.loc.gov/2019050970
LC ebook record available at https://lccn.loc.gov/2019050971

1 2 3 4 5 6 7 8 9 MARQUIS 24 23 22 21 20

For Mom and Dad
who always stood behind me

Contents

PART 3. MORE LIFE

Given the difficulty of mastering any skill, including one as complex as running, the totality of lessons contained in this book should be seen as an introduction on how you might go about improving your stride rather than a complete guide to running with optimal efficiency. For regardless the subject, not only does achieving mastery require enormous space for wonder and exploration, and therefore a tremendous amount of patience and time, but in virtually all cases, it involves a good deal more detailed guidance, instruction, and case examples than any single book can offer. That said, I am confident that the following pages will be a good launching pad to discovery—enough to give you a running start (pun intended) toward deeper learning and lasting improvement.

Prologue

Fewer than twenty-four hours after my formal induction into the Masters' century-old Bagua lineage, I encountered my first reality check. I had just begun practicing when I heard Master Ge's cannon voice reverberating through the park where all the students had gathered that evening.

"That was completely terrible!" he shouted in a tone so filled with disgust that it was as if someone had insulted his entire family.

Somebody is really screwing up, I chuckled to myself as I continued my practice.

"Completely terrible!" Master Ge repeated.

I had never heard him this angry before and felt relieved that I had always been on his good side. Momentarily I imagined Master Ge as a great army general, commanding his troops with incredible tenacity and verve during the heat of the battle. I could hear his voice roaring like a howitzer over the cacophony of exploding gunpowder.

"Terrible!" he repeated a third time.

I wondered how Master Ge's decibel rating would compare to that of an idling metro bus. Obviously, somebody wasn't getting his point, though I didn't immediately see who, since I was several meters away, busily racing through the form. As usual, I was in a hurry to finish up because I wanted to catch the last call at my favorite hole-in-the-wall restaurant down the street. The thought of steamed buns was suddenly making my mouth water.

"Stop!"

I would bet on Master Ge over the bus. Then nothing but a silence so eerie I couldn't resist turning to see what all the commotion had been about.

A momentary glimpse was all I needed to realize that somebody had been insulting his family—the family of Bagua masters who had carried the art through seven generations all the way down to the present moment. Seeing Master Ge squared off like an angry bull, ready to charge in my direction, I felt an instant jolt of both horror and utter disbelief.

Me?

As he brushed me aside and proceeded to mimic what seemed at once to be an exaggerated yet oddly accurate rendition of my movements, I realized my insult. When the masters demonstrate the correct movement and then mimic yours, it's like being handed plastic flowers after having just returned from the botanical garden. My form was indeed a cheap imitation, not simply because I was a relative beginner with thousands of hours of training ahead of me, but moreover because my distraction and lack of enthusiasm had evidently showed. Master Ge had caught me going through the motions, and now that I was representing his lineage, he had no patience for mediocrity.

When I was at the tender age of thirty-two, Master Ge's yelling marked the beginning of a six-hour-a-day, seven-day-a-week training regimen during which I was to discover for the first time in my life what it means to have your heart and mind fully involved. On a cool spring evening in the grit-filled industrial city of Tianjin, China, I was discovering what it means, in other words, to learn.

How to Read This Book

Try to forget everything you've learned as an adult—the things that limit your view of the world, your fears, your prejudices, your preconceptions. Try to rediscover what it is like to be a child with a sense of wonder, and innocence. And don't forget to laugh. Remember, children are strong, they are resilient, they are designed to survive. When you drop them, they tend to bounce.

—TERRY GILLIAM

For those of you who are in a hurry to improve your running and don't have time to go through the philosophy and methodology contained in this book, please skip "Life," "More Life," and "The Rest of Your Life"—that is, part 1, part 3, and the epilogue. I suggest you read part 2, "Practical Matters," or simply go straight to the lessons. There are twenty-seven of them in appendix B.

As you continue to do the lessons regularly, you will begin to feel differences in your body that you may not have felt before, and you will rediscover a certain vibrancy that you long ago forgot existed inside of you. Each new feeling in your body will have the potential to make a profound impact not only in the way you run but in your posture, in your gait, in the way you perform other activities—indeed, in everything involving movement. Each new feeling will, in short, begin to transform the way you live your life.

Some of you will discover that rather than living life, you've been trying to get it over with—as if living were more of a chore than a journey to be experienced fully, deep down inside yourself. In this discovery you will realize that living itself is not the chore, but rather hurrying through life—what I call "not quite living"—that makes our days seem harried and senseless.

For those of you with enough time for the main body of text, be playful—for it is in play that we learn the most. Skip pages and even chapters (I often do when reading books), or start at the end of the book and go backward if you want. Most of all, please slow down and take your time. I hope you will savor the newfound feelings and sensations in your body that come from doing each lesson the way you might savor the sunset, a good piece of chocolate, or perhaps a fine wine. This way you will do three things at once. First, you will actually enjoy yourself. Second, you will learn more. And third, by enjoying and learning more, your running will improve faster. Yes, you read it correctly: by slowing down and enjoying yourself, you will run faster, and you will run faster faster—or in other words, you will improve more rapidly. Conversely, if you plow through the lessons as if they were something to get out of the way, you will not only enjoy them less, but you will improve less—if you improve at all. Going too fast, in other words, will slow you down by hindering your learning.

But to tell the truth, getting you to run faster is not the real reason I wrote this book. There's something much deeper waiting for you between the pages. It exists in the pauses between sentences and in the wondering that will emerge between chapters. It's the gift that you may long ago have forgotten about.

Introduction

Was it possible that modern man might forget his relationship with the rest of the natural world to such a degree that he separated himself from his own heartbeat, wrote poetry only in tune with machines, and was irrevocably cut off from his own heart?

—MARGARET MEAD

I began writing this book in the midst of teaching running classes where instead of showing students how to run, I had them roll around on the floor in slow motion. I mean this quite literally: in my classes, students roll around on the floor. And while they are rolling around, they are encouraged to listen to their bodies. That's all. Simply listen.

The funny thing is when you begin to listen, you start to hear things you haven't heard in a long time, sometimes things that even seem very foreign. It's not that your hearing has been deficient all these years, but more likely that you haven't taken the time to hear. You see, hearing takes time. And listening means giving yourself the time to hear.

What the students heard came from a place deep inside themselves. Voices that had been shut out for a long, long time. Voices that if heeded could put them on a new path for living—a path toward greater power, coordination, balance, flexibility, and pleasure. What students were hearing was the beating of their own heart.

My Not-Quite-Life as a Runner

I myself am not a runner, though I ran track and cross-country in high school and even completed a couple of triathlons before turning twenty. Ironically, now that I no longer train for the sport, I can run faster and with much greater power and ease than when I was twenty-five years younger and running several miles a day. Now that I take my time to roll around on the floor, I have discovered that life arrives when I slow down. It is counterintuitive that speed, power, balance, coordination, and even pleasure can all be linked to slowing down rather than speeding up. How could this be?

What I've discovered in the years since I stopped running is that power does not result from muscling your way through—the "no pain, no gain" sort of approach—but rather by taking your time to listen to what your body is telling you. You actually have to slow down in order to simply hear what your body is saying. There's really no other way.

Your body is speaking constantly. And the biggest difference between the great Olympic runners and the rest of us is not that they are somehow genetically superior, bench press more weight, or have more willpower. It's that they actually hear their bodies. Their hearing is so acute that they often notice the slightest whispers. We teenagers and adults, on the other hand, miss a great deal of what our bodies are saying, and truthfully, we only stop to listen when we can no longer ignore our body's screaming, as in the case of an injury. Anything less and we claim not to hear it. But the truth is we can't hear because we don't listen. We've become caught in a vicious cycle of not listening and thereby corrupting the sensitivity of our hearing.

Imagine going to heavy metal concerts every weekend and standing right next to the loudest speakers. Eventually you will lose the ability to make fine distinctions in sound. You will begin turning the volume on your own stereo higher and higher just to be able to distinguish what you once could effortlessly.

Life for most of us has been some measure of attending heavy metal concerts. The stresses of everyday life have become the noise that blocks out the sounds coming from our bodies. The noisy thoughts in our heads telling us to go faster, work harder, be smarter, look more attractive, be more obedient, be more rebellious, wear this kind of clothing, drive that kind of car, work this kind of job ... all of it plays like the blaring speakers in a concert. We have gotten to the point where we can no longer hear ourselves. In fact, we have given up even listening, by which I mean we have given up listening to our deepest sensations and feelings. We have, in other words, become numb to our own hearts. They go on beating nonetheless, and we go on living, of course, but in a perfunctory way, as if life were something to be endured and survived. We do our best to "kill time" and "get it over with" and in the process, we unwittingly drag ourselves through the prolonged torture of getting through life rather than living it.

Yet through all this, our hearts continue to speak to us. After all these years they haven't forsaken us, but continue to wait for us, hoping one day to be heard. In a sense, they have always been there to guide us to what we once knew. If you follow your heart, you will end up with more than you could ever imagine. But to know what your heart wants, you have to start listening.

Why Start on the Floor?

The reason I often have my students start on the floor is because it reduces the number of distractions bombarding their nervous system. Notice how talking on the phone while driving changes the way you drive. Talking tends to distract you, and in the process your driving suffers.

Each distraction to the nervous system occupies part of your mind, leaving less of it to pay attention to what you want to pay attention to. Getting off your feet frees up the part of your mind that keeps you upright when you're sitting or standing and allows you to pay much more attention to what you're doing. It's like turning down the volume of your stereo so that you can hear the wind blowing outside. In this case what you start to "hear" is the amount of effort you're exerting and the amount of discomfort or comfort you feel. When there is too much noise, you can't sense subtle gradations in either effort or discomfort. Everything is either loud enough to hear over the noise, or else you don't notice it. It's why people don't whisper at rock concerts. And it's why many of us have damaged our bodies over years without even realizing we were doing so. We have turned the volume up so high that we can't hear our bodies speaking. Some of us don't take notice until finally we've herniated a disc, torn ligaments, developed a debilitating physical condition, or collapsed from depression.

Making Sense of Life

The disciplines that have been instrumental in showing me the power of slowing down are Feldenkrais—an ingenious method of learning how to learn—and the timeless Chinese martial arts of Bagua and Taichi. All three involve paying close attention to the sensations and feelings in your body so that you begin to notice how different parts of yourself can work cooperatively rather than in opposition. What we don't realize is that for the most part, we are not working in a unified, cooperative way with our own selves. This means that some parts of us are actually fighting against other parts. It is an internal battle of which we are largely unaware, and the result can be anything from physical pain and injury to those disconcerting moments when something doesn't feel quite right but you can't put your finger on it. It can be subtle, like a barely noticeable tightness in your chest, or it can bear down on you and feel as if sandbags have been draped over your shoulders.

Improving sensory awareness is like dropping the sandbags, so to speak, thereby allowing you to move with more precision and power, which in turn can lead to profound improvements in the way you run. More importantly, improving awareness can lead to greater enjoyment of the activity of running itself.

PART 1 LIFE

(You may want to skip this part if you are in a hurry.)

1

Running (and Other Things We Want to Get Over With)

I open my eyes and don't know where I am or who I am. Not all that unusual—I've spent half my life not knowing.

—ANDRE AGASSI, *OPEN: AN AUTOBIOGRAPHY*

Years ago when I was a runner, my favorite part about running was sitting down after a race. Actually, it was virtually the only thing I liked about the sport, since I found it to be torturously painful, and at times dreadfully boring. Obviously I didn't run because I enjoyed it. Yet the motivation to continue had to come from somewhere, and in my case, a lot of self-esteem was wrapped up in doing well, being "fit," looking good, and trying to be something that I wasn't. Like most teenagers—indeed, like most adults as well—I spent a lot of time trying to be rather than being, and believe it or not, this takes a lot of energy. As you will see later, trying to be requires forcefully restraining what is. It is as if two beings are inhabiting the same body: one being, and the other trying to be. In athletics, such internal conflict stifles speed, strength, coordination, balance, and agility. Outside of athletics, such internal conflict stifles everything from creativity to spontaneity to your ability to deal with stress. So, where my trying to be made me run harder, it simultaneously stifled my running and my life outside of running.

I am not alone.

If you observe the posture of most people while they're running, you will likely feel discomfort in your own body. Compare this to the feeling you have when you watch Olympic runners glide down the track. You can actually sense their power and effortlessness. It looks so easy. So why isn't it easy for the rest of us?

Running may be unpleasant or otherwise less than joyful for the same reason many of us find it uninteresting: we can't feel our own bodies. By this, I mean we have a general sense of effort and strain and maybe even endorphins flowing into our bloodstream from time to time, but we don't know what it feels like to have our entire selves working together in unison.

The primary difference between Olympic runners and the rest of us is not that they possess superior strength, endurance, or willpower, but that they aren't busy sabotaging themselves. Unlike many of us, virtually all of their effort goes toward their intended purpose: moving forward swiftly. Much of our effort, on the other hand, inadvertently goes toward slowing us down. It's like hitting the brakes and the accelerator at the same time, which may explain why our engine feels like it's straining.

Of course, acting this way does not make sense. And the reason it doesn't make sense is because we cannot sense what we are doing. We are unaware that we are literally fighting ourselves with every step.

Turning the Doorknob

When you see somebody who can't type, they start with two fingers. If they go on typing like that, they won't gradually use ten fingers. They will get better and better at using this terrible method. The hands move very fast like a couple of mad hens. But they never develop a good technique and the result is that typing is always a strain and an effort.

—TREVOR LEGGETT, *THE DRAGON MASK*

In modern society, grinding and straining have become the norm by which we measure our lives. Running is simply one aspect of this. "I guess I wasn't meant to be a good runner," I might say, or perhaps, "Running isn't meant to be fun." I might begin to think that I'm not working hard enough. Doctors might tell me that aches and pains are simply part of the aging process (They won't say, however, that self-destruction is part of the aging process). Specialists might say that my knees (insert any body part you like—whatever part that hurts) weren't designed for such pounding and advise me to stop. They might even say that no knees or backs or necks were designed for such pounding. Of course they might be right, but has it occurred to them what the source of the pounding is?

We are like a person in front of a door, pushing on the door, kicking it, pounding on it, knocking our heads against it, and doing everything but taking the easiest approach: simply turning the knob.

I know this because I am one of those who went for the conventional approach, enduring years of strenuous training in high school that continued for a couple of years afterward when I competed in triathlons. Though I ran on a State Championship cross-country team my senior year, and later placed well in triathlons, I almost never found running to be particularly easy or enjoyable. With rare exceptions, running remained drudgery and a major chore that I naturally did not look forward to. And it was symbolic for how I lived the rest of my life, slogging through what I thought was an endless struggle to attain that ever-elusive feeling of success.

Virtually all of us are striving for success, and consequently, many of us end up doing things we really don't want to do. For those who suffer, this book is especially for you.

Some of us, on the other hand, spend our days doing mainly what we want to do. Some of us, for example, run because we are entirely in love with the activity. For those who love running, this book is especially for you. Regardless of how much you suffer or how much you enjoy running, there is always time to slow down.

2

The Hurried Runner (a.k.a. "The Bulldozer")

Instant coffee is punishment for people who are in too much of a hurry.

—ALAN WATTS

In order to stop fighting ourselves, and thereby unintentionally slowing ourselves down, we must be aware that we are actually doing it. And in order to be aware of it, we need to literally feel it. Feeling leads to awareness, and awareness leads to more speed, power, and agility.

But how could the solution be so simple? you may be thinking. *If it were that easy, we would all be great runners ... wouldn't we?*

Yes, we would, but we would have to reverse all the years of assimilation of our "hurry-up" culture in order for this to happen.

Hurrying is a symptom of modern society's fixation on accomplishment. It is a constant preoccupation that I need to be somewhere other than where I am, doing something other than what I am doing at this moment, being someone other than who I am. It is a major reason why many of us are not fully present in daily life, our attention wandering far away from us—into the past, or future.

You may think that running and walking are the perfect activities for people in a hurry. You may think that the way to improve is to hurry more—to use what I call the "do it faster, get it over with" approach. And you will sense such attitudes in people scurrying past you on the street. Something about them says, "Don't get in my way because I'm in a hurry!" Interestingly, if you really pay attention, it is not their speed that cues you into their hurriedness. They may not even be traveling any faster than anyone else. There's something else—a certain characteristic that you can't put your finger on, but that nonetheless registers as a feeling of dis-ease in your own body.

The renowned Bagua master Guoliang Ge used to say to me, "Your form should be beautiful. It should look unhurried, graceful, easy, and effortless. It should not be painful to watch, putting observers into distress. If you put people in distress, you are not doing Bagua." When you watched Master Ge in action, you got a sense of awesome power, resulting from grace and effortlessness rather than a gnashing of teeth and straining of muscles. Because he was never in a hurry, his movements remained fluid and powerful rather than choppy and tension-ridden. What was more surprising to observers was that his unhurried attitude gave him tremendous speed and precision. Even highly trained martial artists half his age could not match his quickness and agility. When they made contact with him, they would, in a flash, find themselves lying on their backs.

If You Can't Feel Yourself, Then You Can't Feel Yourself Feeling Good

In well-made chocolate, the sweetness should highlight the cacao's natural complexity and bitterness the way it can when you add small amounts to a cup of good espresso. Excessive amounts of sugar will bring a big burst of sweetness and then ... nothing. This hollowness is what makes the lack of flavor in low-grade chocolate so glaringly apparent. No wonder people eat whole bars of bad chocolate in a manner of minutes.

—ARI WEINZWEIG, *ZINGERMAN'S GUIDE TO GOOD EATING*

In a world where "time is money," emphasis on speed tends to sabotage speed. It may seem like a contradiction, but it isn't. Great athletes, dancers, musicians, writers, scientists, educators and martial artists all know this. To them it is obvious. Albert Einstein never said, "If I don't finish the General Theory of Relativity by five o'clock, my mother will never love me again." Had the great Bagua and Taichi masters not given themselves time to make new discoveries, they would not have become masters, and consequently, instead of their art and insight, we would have women and men, like us, too busy to take notice of life.

Hurrying, in one sense, is commanding yourself to do something without paying attention to how you do it. This is why most people become rather clumsy and careless when they are rushed. They are unaware of where they are, say, losing balance, or gripping excessively with their hands. This is because most people, when commanded to do anything, either by themselves or by others, will tend to strain and carry anxiety into whatever it is that they are doing. They will say, "Last time wasn't good enough, so this time I must try harder." Of course, they may not say it audibly, or even consciously think it, but something about them is screaming, "Faster! Harder! More effort!"

The question is, who is really in command? Or to put it another way, what part of you is trying, and what part is being tried? As you have surely noticed, your body has been answering this question all your life. It speaks to you through the tension you may feel in your neck and shoulders, the pain you may feel in your joints, the strain you may feel in your jaw, the tightening you may feel in your throat and chest, the tiredness you may experience when you are engaging in a particular activity. Its voice is also the feeling of openness in your chest, the ease you feel at certain times when everything seems to be going right, the joy you feel when partaking in activities you like. Of course, when you spend most of your time doing what you don't want to do, you may even forget how to feel good. You may reach a point early in life when fully letting go and feeling pleasure becomes very difficult. Strange as it may sound, most people I encounter have difficulty fully enjoying life because they have forgotten how to feel themselves. And if they can't feel themselves, they can't feel themselves feeling good.

And this brings us back to hurrying: when we hurry and thereby command ourselves to do something, what are we in fact doing? Do we really get the job done faster? Is it done well?

At each and every moment of our life, we have the possibility to discover something new. Great athletes know this intuitively and make use of this possibility in their work and often in their play—in fact their work often looks like play. Children too understand this intuitively, which is why they tend to laugh frequently and learn much faster than adults.

Each infant, in fact, has an intimate relationship with discovery. Infants are constantly at play, discovering new movements and new relationships with the world. They take complete initiative for their own learning, and if they did not, they would never crawl, much less stand up on their own two feet.[1]

We Are Unaware That We Are Unaware

If you consider that there are an infinite number of ways to hurry, then looking at how you hurry can give you clues about what you're actually doing with your body. When you are in a hurry, notice how much you see in front of you. How much of your environment do you notice through your eyes, ears, nose, touch? What happens to your breathing?

---

[1] In our culture, we often prod and push children to stand and walk before they are ready. We hurry them, in other words, to do what they would normally do if left to their own devices. "When parents have greater respect for the learning process of the young human being, for whom everything is strange and new, and they restrain their expressions of approval at the first signs of success—especially with regard to standing and walking, which are accomplishments vulnerable to distortion—the child can ripen in her own time and arrive at the ability to stand when she is better prepared and trained, and capable of continuing to refine the process as well. The child receives a firm foundation for her entire life, not only in the alignment of the spine, not only in the ease and comfort with which she relates to standing and to physical activity in general, but also in the sense that she has a better chance of growing and going through the obstacles of life forever free of having to earn love through actions which she does or does not perform. Such a lucky child could believe that being born is sufficient reason for being loved." Ruthy Alon, *Mindful Spontaneity: Lessons in the Feldenkrais Method* (Berkeley, CA: North Atlantic Books, 1996), 229.

In general, the more hurried we are, the more we behave like the person who is so thoroughly frantic in looking for his car keys that he doesn't notice them sitting right in front of him. Were he to pause and breathe, he would see more of the complete picture. Being hurried, however, his vision will have narrowed sufficiently such that he will waste more time looking for what is staring him in the face. It seems ridiculous, but this is how most of us behave. We are unaware of the alternatives. And we are unaware that we are unaware.

John's Story[2]

Not only do we have to be good at waiting, we have to love it. Because waiting is not waiting, it is life.

—JOSH WAITZKIN, *THE ART OF LEARNING*

John was an avid salsa dancer who arrived in class one day complaining of chronic back and neck pain. He had come not to run faster, but simply in the hope of finding a way to alleviate his suffering.

I started the students on their backs with some gentle rolling that allowed them to, among other things, discover and create connections between their feet, hips, and spine. After a few minutes, John stopped and covered his eyes with his hands.

I had noticed that despite frequent suggestions to slow down and pay attention, he continued to race along hurriedly, as if afraid of falling behind. Rather than paying attention to himself, his eyes never left me as I walked around the room giving instructions. Meanwhile, his birdlike movements

---

[2] John is, in fact, a fictional character, but infused with a good bit of nonfiction. To be specific, he is a conglomeration of people I have met, and in some cases, gotten to know quite well. In many ways, John reminds me of the way I used to behave when under stress … or maybe the way I still behave under stress (as my wife likes to remind me).

were done with a certainty that I see in many new students. It is a certainty that says, "Okay, I did it. Now, what's next?"[3]

Certainty, whether in words or movement, not only communicates an attitude, but more importantly, solidifies beliefs and habitual movement patterns. When I am certain, I am saying to myself, "This is the way I do it," which is often simply another way of saying, "My way is the one right way to do it." If you have ever watched a political debate, or read a how-to book (for example, a book on running), then you know what I'm talking about. Because certainty avoids wavering, it can be very useful for getting the job done. But what happens if there is more than one way? What if there are other ways that actually work better?

The Power of Awareness

When I was in school, most of us were busy trying to get the right answers. We were, in other words, trying to be right. But trying to be something also means trying not to be something else. What, you might wonder, were we trying not to be?

Like all of us, John perceived a world filtered through his assumptions, one of which happened to be, "Gotta move fast and get it done." Part and parcel of this assumption was a chronic clenching of his jaw, locking of his knees, holding of his breath, and tightening of his fingers. He had unconsciously chosen these strategies to represent his "rightness."

John is not alone.

Most of us unwittingly choose such strategies to uphold our own rightness. And hold up we do, as if carrying sandbags over our heads. By this, I am not saying that holding ourselves "right"—or to put it another way, being self-righteous—is necessarily a bad thing, but rather that doing so may not always be in our best interest. Living in Los Angeles, for example, I might assume that I'm "right" to drive on the right side of the road. But if I unconsciously carry this "rightness" to London or Tokyo, I'll find myself facing in the wrong direction.

---

[3] Of course, the answer is, "nothing." For once you have canceled out the present moment, that is all you are left with.

Were we to slow down and become conscious of it, we would realize that we always have a choice and that it might be a good idea to check the local traffic rules, so to speak. If we are married to the agenda of being right, on the other hand, we may never see the choice, rushing instead into oncoming traffic and wondering why everyone else is driving in the "wrong" direction.

Our Unfamiliarity with Slowness

Eventually John slowed down enough to begin noticing his own patterns. One of the first things he noticed while lying on his back was that he got dizzy and sometimes nauseous whenever he slowed down. His nervous system—and his system was indeed nervous—was so used to going at warp speed that gentle, slow movement had become something entirely alien and uncomfortable.

As a salsa dancer you might think that John would have no problem performing slow movements. The assumption here is that slow movements are easier to perform than faster ones and that swing dancing with its fast, whirling steps would be more likely to make you dizzy or nauseous than lying on your back and gently rocking side to side. Yet in a culture that places a premium on going faster, it is more likely that its inhabitants are more accustomed to scurrying about at high speed than slowly and methodically exploring movement. In such a culture, anxiety runs rampant and people's movements tend to be linear, choppy, and clumsy, rather than smooth, graceful, and coordinated. If you consider that learning occurs through your sensory system, what we are teaching ourselves in our compulsion to "get it done" is how to be anxious, uncoordinated, and clumsy. What we present to our minds is a version of balance and equilibrium that is ironically unbalanced and un-equilibrated. When imbalance and disequilibrium have become the norm, moving toward balance and equilibrium can initially provide a disturbing contrast to the nervous system.

3

What Does It Mean to "Slow Down"?

Newton's patience was limitless. Truth, he said much later, was "the offspring of silence and meditation."

—JAMES GLEICK, *ISAAC NEWTON*

The greatest improvements in power, speed, coordination, agility, and balance will occur when we slow down enough to become aware of the proverbial sandbags we are carrying. Slowing down allows us to become aware of what we were previously unaware of.

If this is the case, what does it mean to "slow down"?

The answer seems obvious, yet if we all knew, I would never have written this book, and you probably wouldn't be reading it.

I have noticed in my years of teaching that when I ask new students to slow down, all of them, with very little exception, continue to move very quickly. Their idea of slowing down and mine are obviously not the same.

How slow is slow enough?

This question can be answered by another question: how slow do you need to go in order to discover something new? Consider that slowing down is simply a tool by which you can become aware of things that you were not previously aware of. And what you are not aware of is precisely what keeps you from running with more power.

This means that there is no set speed for the word *slow*. The appropriate speed is determined by what it takes to feel and sense and therefore experience more at any given moment. And since circumstances change from moment to moment, pacing needs to change as well. In this regard, slowing down could translate to an endless search for the ideal pace for increasing awareness at any given moment. It is endless not because you never find what's appropriate, but because every moment is a new moment. The searching alone is what allows you to become more aware.

Another way of looking at speed is to view it from the standpoint of receiving information. The human nervous system is designed to handle an enormous amount of information—so much so that neuroscientists are still astonished by its processing abilities. Yet, while the amount that it can process appears to be almost limitless, the pace at which it can receive, or in other words, take in new information, remains limited. If too much information is dumped onto the nervous system at once, it will be lost. This is because entry into the nervous system is akin to getting water to pass through a bottleneck. If you attempt to pour a bucket of water all at once into a bottle, almost all of it will end up as a puddle on the floor. Similarly, if you present your nervous system with too much new information at once—something that tends to happen when you are moving quickly—the information will be spilled into the ether, so to speak, and you will have forsaken the opportunity for learning and improvement.

Riding the Bullet Train

Imagine riding a bullet train and trying to observe objects that are within a few feet the tracks. If you're going too fast, all you will see is a blur, possibly making you dizzy, or even nauseous. When going at top speed—say, 200 miles an hour—nothing will be discernible. If the train slows down to 190 miles an hour, you will still see nothing but a blur. While it is true that your speed was just reduced by 10 miles an hour, the picture you are seeing will not be much clearer, if at all. Even if the train keeps decreasing its speed, it will take a considerable amount of slowing down before anything close to the window is discernible from anything else—that is, before you begin to even vaguely recognize what it is that you are seeing. Quite likely everything between 190 and 20 miles an hour will be too blurry to tell. Perhaps at 20 you will start to be able to discern gross differences. One moment, for example, you may think that you just passed a four-legged animal rather than a human. You may assume it's a dog because of its size, but truthfully, it could have been a leopard, a goat, or a large piñata, considering that all you saw was a blurry mass with four leg-like attachments. The next moment you might know that you just passed a car rather than an elephant, but you still won't know the make or model.

When you approach 15 miles an hour, things get much clearer relative to 20 miles an hour. But you will still miss details. Was that a man or a woman? Was the person wearing glasses? What did that sign say? As you approach slower speeds, even more will become discernible. And it is only when you are on the verge of stopping that you may finally be able to read the print on a flyer, or notice the stitching on someone's sweater, sense the curve of a man's chin, notice the cracks in the cement, gaze at a spiderweb, and possibly even locate the spider in it.

In our fast-paced world, we are moving like a bullet train going at top speed—that is to say, way too fast for our nervous system to keep up with. In this manner we are depriving our nervous system of new information and therefore preventing ourselves from learning. Yet we continue to wonder why every time we look out the window we see nothing but blurry images. We may occasionally slow down, but have we slowed down enough so that we can actually perceive more of the world? And herein lies the catch: Even though going from 200 to 190 miles an hour is indeed slowing down, and going from 190 to 50 miles an hour is slowing down even more, it isn't nearly enough to catch what is right outside the window (despite the fact that going from 200 to 50 miles an hour is a whopping 75 percent decrease in speed!).

We are all conductors of our own bullet train. By not slowing down enough to make distinctions, we continue to bar new information from entering our nervous system, and this leaves us repeating the same old habits that have prevented us from improving in the first place.

By slowing down enough so that we can discern differences, we let in new information, and this in turn allows us to move away from our habits. In the case of movement, discernment comes through sensing and feeling. Can you, for example, sense how much effort it takes to lift your left leg compared to your right? Do you begin to tighten your chest or hold your breath as you slowly lifted your leg? Do you begin to wobble?

As you slow down more, you will begin to notice subtler and subtler changes. Like seeing the spider in the web, you will feel places where you were holding unnecessarily, but wouldn't have noticed had you been going faster. You will feel parts that have been overused and others that have been asleep and therefore not doing the work that they were meant to do. You will literally feel yourself in ways that you have not felt before. And it is in this increased sensitivity to your own movements that you will begin to run with greater power and ease.

4

The Art of Learning: You Already Have Everything You Need

Normal adults never stop to think about such concepts as space and time. These are things children ask about. My secret is I remained a child. I always asked the simplest questions. I ask them still.

—ALBERT EINSTEIN

For me, teaching running classes that involve little to no actual running is not contradictory, though it is anathema to the way I was "taught" to run. You see, most education is a process of a teacher, coach, parent, expert, or even advertising agency trying to superimpose "correctness" or "rightness" on top of you. In film photography, when you superimpose one image on top of another, the original negative is not transformed in any way. This means that while the projected image may look different, it is only because you covered up the original with something else. Similarly, you could say that conventional education is to a large degree about covering something up, and unfortunately, that something just happens to be you.

The result of all of this superimposition is that, as we grow older, we become less and less aware of the original lying beneath everything else. This is based on our mostly unconscious and long-held assumption that the original is not good enough—otherwise why would we bother covering it up? But what if the assumption is totally inaccurate? What if buried beneath all the layers was a quintessentially curious and exploratory being—a consummate learner, in other words, just waiting to be uncovered? If we looked at it this way, then all of our efforts might be akin to a museum curator trying to add highlights to the *Mona Lisa* in an attempt to make her more mysterious and beautiful, or a park ranger trying to bulldoze the Grand Canyon trying to make it grander.

Superimposition, though the predominant force in conventional education, is simply one of an infinite number of approaches to learning and improvement. Another possibility is a different sort of interaction that allows for the transformation of the student by drawing out what is already inside. Thus, instead of the teacher superimposing on the student and the student being taught by the teacher, the interaction becomes a process of discovery through self-discovery.

If we look in the dictionary, we find that the roots of education as discovery through self-discovery go back to antiquity. The English word *education* comes from the Latin word *educare*, which means "to draw forth." Contrary to what education has come to mean, its root presupposes that everything you require is already inside you. The seeds of knowledge and wisdom, in other words, lie dormant in your very being. All you need is to find a process that allows them to sprout forth. When the learning process involves a teacher, I call it *educaring* because it is distinct from conventional educating.[1] In educaring the teacher helps to draw out the student's innate intelligence, and in doing so, the innate intelligence of both begin to emerge. Unlike in conventional education, the teacher and student are then

---

[1] I am borrowing the term *educare* from the magnificent early childhood educator Magda Gerber. The enormous success of her educational—or perhaps more accurately stated, *educaring*—centers gives potent testimony to the notion that true learning does not occur by having someone, namely a teacher, impose something on someone else, namely a student.

involved in an interactive learning process of give and take, more akin to a symbiotic dance than a covering up of one by the other. Rather than the teacher superimposing and the student being superimposed upon, teacher and student engage in a cooperative project of uncovering layers from the original, so to speak.

As you may have already suspected, learning does not require the physical presence of a teacher (if it did, there would be little point in independently exploring the lessons in this book) even though it can sometimes be very helpful. This is because in *educaring*, a teacher—or *educarer*—serves mainly as an observer and guide to assist in the student's own learning process. Thus, rather than doling out prepackaged information, as is the norm in a conventional classroom, the *educarer* creates an environment whereby the student can draw on her own resources to discover on her own. Obviously, if you, the reader, are willing, patient, and observant, you can and will fulfill this role on your own. In fact, you may have already taught—or *educared*—yourself if you skipped ahead to the lessons. The degree to which, upon trying a lesson, you explored new possibilities, began to notice those moments when you deviated from the given constraints, and all the while, observed your feelings and sensations, is the degree to which you began to uncover your own innate intelligence.

Wonder

Uncovering your own innate intelligence—or, in a word, learning—is simpler than you might expect. It involves two components: wonder and observation. If you want a direct experience of this process, try Lesson 27, "Where Does My Arm Begin?" before reading further.

Those of you who explored Lesson 27 may have noticed that just by wondering, your state of attention began to shift, making it possible to feel and therefore uncover more of yourself. The state of wonder is optimum for learning because it works to uncover layers of superimposed thoughts and movement habits that have been preventing you from sensing and feeling. Wondering and observing detach you from your habits, and in the process, actually sharpen your ability to sense and feel.

Knowing this, it may not surprise you that wonder is a state used by wine tasters to fully appreciate the impact that wine has on their senses. By cultivating their sense of smell and taste over time, wine tasters can differentiate flavors to extraordinarily subtle degrees.

What about other disciplines? Consider that wine is just a metaphor for life and that our bodies are like fine wines waiting to be fully sensed and enjoyed. Bagua and Taichi masters are the great "samplers" of the human body, being able to differentiate extremely fine degrees of muscular effort the way wine tasters differentiate flavors and aromas. The masters can in fact discern body alignment and muscle tension to such minute levels that they are able to make themselves as heavy as a boulder in one instant, and as light and ethereal as smoke in the next.

If It Ain't Broke ...

Imagination is as effortless as perception, unless we think it might be "wrong," which is what our education encourages us to believe. Then we experience ourselves as "imagining," as "thinking up an idea," but what we're really doing is faking up the sort of imagination we think we ought to have.

—KEITH JOHNSTONE, *IMPRO: IMPROVISATION AND THE THEATRE*

Educaring posits that there is actually nothing wrong with you and therefore nothing that needs to be fixed. It also assumes that learning occurs naturally, or in other words, when you are not trying to learn. Contrary to popular belief, trying to learn not only does little to help the process, but often blocks it. Attempting to do something that would happen anyway—that is, without your insistence—is like trying to aid a dolphin by attaching fins to its tail and scuba gear to its back.

Learning, in other words, has less to do with trying to make something happen, and more to do with allowing it to occur. The process of allowing new ideas and possibilities to arrive, rather than impatiently trying to force them into existence, is the same one that many great athletes use. By not fixating on achievement, the great ones actually achieve much more. By trusting the process, and not trying to make something happen, they know that something profound will arrive.

5

Intention

Why is observation so difficult? Because we have the tendency to see what we "know," what we believe in, rather than what is happening in front of our eyes.... We must learn to see as a baby sees—new.

—MAGDA GERBER

If you consider that all of us mastered the act of running sometime in child-hood, how do we account for our differences in speed, power, and fluidity? How do we account for world-class runners being world-class and the rest of us not being world-class? When we watch great runners on television, there is normally some quality in their stride that we would like to possess but that we can't quite identify. And because we can't put our finger on what they are doing to run with such power and grace, we have little choice but to simply continue running the way we have always run. That is, we have little choice but to simply practice our particular manner of running.

So we practice. And we practice more. And we try harder. And in the end, our endurance, willpower, and even times may improve, but the way we run is still basically the same. By practicing what we already know, we haven't learned anything fundamentally new.

This is not to say that the way we run is wrong, or that we are to blame for our lack of learning. Rather, what I am saying is that compared to learning better mechanics, working on endurance and willpower will do little if anything to help us understand what it is that makes great runners run with such phenomenal speed and power. Put another way, short of learning more mechanically efficient ways to use our bodies, we may improve our endurance, but we will not improve the way we run. And it is primarily the way Olympic athletes run that gives them the speed and power that we so desire.

The Crucial Difference

Over the years I have noticed that most expert advice on improving running covers two basic formulas: (1) following the latest training regimen, and (2) working on technique. In advocating these, however, the experts unwittingly make a false assumption: practice what you already know and you will get better.

This statement is false because neither changing your training regimen nor following technical advice addresses the learning that must take place if you are to run with more mechanical efficiency. And the statement is unwittingly false because technical advice, while attempting to address body mechanics, is often too difficult to accurately follow (more on this in chapter 10, "Following Instructions: Where Do My Knees Begin?").

Surprisingly, even the simplest-sounding instructions are normally too complicated, vague, or ambiguous for people to follow with any accuracy. The result, then, is that even when heeding the experts, we usually end up practicing what we already know—that is, we end up practicing all of the mechanical habits that have prevented us from fundamentally improving in the first place.

Of course, it can still be beneficial for us to work on endurance and willpower. But endurance and willpower are still separate issues from body mechanics. And there are strict limitations as to how far you can improve if you are not addressing the latter. These limitations are why mechanical efficiency, or to put it more simply, *power*, is the crucial difference separating great runners from good ones and good ones from their average counterparts.

Are You Motivated by One and Only One Intention?

One way to understand the vital role that mechanics plays in running is to examine the role of intention. The critical difference between Olympic runners and most of the rest of us is that for Olympians, virtually all of their effort goes toward their intention of moving forward swiftly. Most of us, on the other hand, unwittingly devote a large amount of effort toward contradicting ourselves, thereby making our bodies heavier and slower. In fact, most of what people call "inability," whether in running or any other discipline, could be thought of as ability that has been unconsciously sabotaged. This is to say that anything less than highly efficient movement—a powerful stride, in the case of running—has little if anything to do with genetics, endurance, fitness level, or willpower, and everything to do with what we unwittingly do to block ourselves. Yes, you read it correctly: our lack of power is our own doing—or perhaps, more aptly put, it is our undoing.

Stated another way, lack of power is more a result of conflicted intention, otherwise known as self-sabotage, rather than any of the other factors previously mentioned. Contrary to its conventional definition, intention is not cut-and-dried, but rather something that can actually be clarified and refined. The difficulty in realizing this is that much of our intention lies beneath the level of consciousness, so we are only aware of what remains above the surface, in our conscious mind. This means that while we may have one conscious intention—say, to run as fast as possible—beneath the surface, there may be many other conflicting, parasitic forces. Unfortunately, the conflict plays out in our bodies as if we are at war with ourselves, the possible result being postural defects, mechanical inefficiency, pain, or injury.

If, for example, we examine how the average person runs, we will discover places where she unconsciously collapses her body. These are places where muscles seem to be asleep. As this is going on, parts of her that are not sleeping have to perform double duty to make up for the parts that are sleeping. But mechanical efficiency relies on all parts working cooperatively, and in unison. Not only is the sleeping part not participating, it's getting in the way, like dead weight. So our average runner has to carry it around like a sack of gravel.

Examples of conflicted intention can be observed not just in running but in daily life, where many of us are wanting to stay alert, pay attention, and do good work, yet remain unable to do so even with the aid of drugs, the threat of punishment, or the reward of something such as a paycheck. The fact that even those who are considered productive rely on caffeine or nicotine to get them through their average day (and perhaps sleeping pills to get them through their average night) indicates that even the best of us are often burdened with conflicted intention. This is to say, when we are unable to perform as smoothly as we would like, something is happening beneath the level of conscious intention that is driving us down. Thus, to go back to the previous example, if our conscious intention to stay alert and perform well does not match the fact that we are often sleepy, apathetic, and distracted, then our unconscious intention is probably doing something to undermine our efforts.

Unintended Self-Sabotage

From a purely neuromuscular point of view, unrefined intention is manifest in two ways. First, it appears in the phenomenon I described above in which parts of us are habitually sleeping. In this case, certain muscles remain hypotonic, or overly flaccid when at rest, and underused when performing an action. Second, it appears in what somatic pioneer Moshe Feldenkrais called parasitic muscle contractions, whereby certain muscles remain hypertonic, or overly contracted, when at rest, and overused when performing an action.

In either case, unrefined intention acts like the defense of the opposing team in a football game in that it diverts force to where you don't want it to go. In football, the running back wants to take the ball straight down the field to score, but every member of the defense is trying to stop her. Each is a barrier around which she must travel in order to move forward.

From a biomechanical standpoint, I am the host organism to my own parasitic muscle contractions, all of which serve to both absorb and misdirect force, and thereby disrupt my coordination, balance, and strength. Even though my conscious intention is to move forward, some of my unconscious intention drives me in other directions. Aside from the extra burden of work this places on me, some of the force inevitably ends up getting stuck in my joints, causing torsion, shearing, and compression, otherwise known as undue wear and tear. At the same time, because parasitic tension constricts the flow of everything from blood, lymph, and oxygen to various waste materials, a good portion of my effort is not only inadvertently self-defeating on a biomechanical level, but self-destructive on an organic and cellular level.

The Two Principles of Movement

Parasitic contractions in any part of your body will inhibit the smooth translation of force throughout your entire body. Chronically tense backs, shoulders, and necks, for example, inhibit the fluid and powerful strides that we see in world-class athletes. Even tight fingers or a tight jaw can to some degree inhibit powerful and fluid movement in the rest of the body. This is why many boxers keep their hands loose and only clench their fist at the last moment, just as they are making impact.

To understand how parasitic contractions sabotage movement, we need to look into the following two fundamental principles of movement: (1) for every action, there is an equal and opposite reaction, and (2) your mind controls your muscles.

The first principle, sometimes known as the action-reaction law, comes from the preeminent scientist Isaac Newton. When we apply his principle to biomechanics, we discover that contracting any muscle in your body automatically pulls your center of mass, and therefore your entire body, in a certain direction. This means that your entire body is influenced by every single contraction of every single muscle fiber contained in it, which makes obvious sense when you think about it. Muscles pull, and that pull must have a direction. Of course, we need pulling in order to move about. But what if we are pulling in unwanted directions and consequently pulling ourselves off-balance and therefore off-course? Then we have to expend added energy to keep ourselves in balance and on course so that we don't end up falling, or traveling in the wrong direction.

Every movement you make involves your entire body. Even if you only intend to move your left pinky, its movement is part of a larger neurological pattern encompassing your entire body. This is because muscles that are not obviously involved in moving your pinky are still active even if you are not aware of it. Each muscle fiber is, in fact, constantly firing to one degree or another. A muscle that is perpetually overworking and held within confined ranges of motion tends to be chronically short and tense. In contrast, its antagonist—that is, the muscle or muscle group pulling the joint in the opposite direction—is in a sense perpetually dormant, making it chronically long and flaccid. Of course, muscles do not contract by themselves. They are connected to a brain and nervous system that issue the executive orders.

What differentiates Olympic runners from others is that they are able to control their 630-odd muscles in such a manner as to optimize efficiency in their stride. This means the shortening and lengthening of each and every muscle in their body is coordinated in such a way that they are able to minimize resistance and maximize propulsion. In being more accurate, precise, and therefore effective in controlling their muscles, Olympic runners exhibit far fewer parasitic muscle contractions and thus far less unconscious self-sabotage.

Moving with speed, strength, and agility requires coordinating all of the muscular contractions throughout your entire body in a precise fashion. No muscle can pull too much or too little at any given moment. To accomplish such precision, your brain and nervous system have to monitor each and every muscle cell in order to adjust its pulling to just the right amount of contractive force at just the right time. Quite an extraordinary feat, if you consider how many millions of muscle cells inhabit the human body. If speed, strength, and agility are proportional to how precisely your brain and nervous system coordinate the contraction of each and every muscle cell in your body, then sharpening your mind and removing parasitic intention should play a major role in training.

The question, then, is how do you sharpen your mind so that it is able to coordinate your muscles more precisely?

6

Have You Lost Your Senses?

Our initiatory rite begins at the moment of birth when, typically, we take the child away from the mother and put it in a sterile environment. The rite continues with early weaning and the taboo on sucking, and culminates in the drama of toilet training. These three separative efforts are initiated much sooner in our culture than in others. They help to create a continuum of self-imagery which denies the discontinuous, pulsating life of the body. They lead to acceptance of an artificial schedule, a socially imposed rhythm that kills individual rhythmicity. Wake up at 8. Brush your teeth at 8:05. Eat your breakfast at 8:10 and out the door. Catch the bus at 8:20. Go to school 9 to 5.

—STANLEY KELEMAN, *YOUR BODY SPEAKS ITS MIND*

For three hundred years Western civilization has taken a reductionistic view on humanity, behaving as though the human mind were nothing more than gray matter sloshing between our ears. We have been acting, in other words, as if the gelatinous stew resting in our cranium operates independently from the rest of our body and is therefore capable of functioning normally without any connection to feeling, sensing, or emoting. In this manner, our emotionless Spock-like mind controls our machinelike body: our brain, which is like a test tube of biochemicals to be titrated, manipulates our body, which is like a collection of joints to be resurfaced and "parts" to be stretched, replaced, cauterized, radiated, or simply extracted. This way of viewing the mind and body treats the human whole as a collection of discrete parts that function with little or no relation to each other. A foot problem, for example, is generally not thought to be related to the way you use your knees and hips, much less the way you carry your head. In this case, the foot is considered the sole cause (no pun intended) of its problems. As a result, surgeons may saw off bunions, fuse joints, reconstruct arches, and prescribe pain-killers, but nobody seems willing to address the elephant in the room: how do the mind and body connected to that foot relate to its use or misuse? And, just as important, how does the movement of that foot relate to the use or misuse of the rest of the body?

In reality, the health and performance of each and every part of your body depends on the performance of each and every other part. Your overall health and performance, in other words, is related to whether or not your "parts" are working cooperatively.

Mind-Body Unity

When people hear the word *measuring instrument,* they will likely picture digital scales, calipers, voltmeters, or perhaps some high-tech device with flashing lights. As a runner you might picture a heart-rate monitor, pedometer, or calorie counter. Few, however, will consider the most powerful instrument of them all, perhaps because it is hidden inside each and every one of us, theoretically not for sale.

Even with major advances in technology over the last half-century, engineers have yet to design a bipedal machine capable of walking, much less running, with the power, speed, agility and elegance of humans. And the enormity of the task makes it unlikely that they ever will. As we shall see in chapter 10 ("Following Instructions: Where Do My Knees Begin?"), the mechanics of human movement are, in fact, so complex that they require an instrument far more powerful than the most advanced supercomputer to govern them. To achieve the kind of elegant and powerful movement that we see in Olympic athletes requires a mind that is not Spock-like, and a body that is not machinelike. It requires a mind and body that are one and the same.

Not surprisingly, the reductionistic way of viewing life has led to people moving more and more like machines—that is, in a choppy and linear rather than smooth and spiraling manner. The majority of contraptions in health clubs, for example, are designed to isolate body parts so that rather than creating fluid full-body movement, they inadvertently train you to move in a jerky, robotic fashion. While this may be useful for increasing muscle mass, it can have the unfortunate effect of making you less coordinated and agile.

It is of note that prior to the introduction of reductionistic principles, people from both East and West did not separate the mind and the body. Perhaps this is why, for millennia, the Chinese have used the same character to represent both mind and heart. According to the Chinese, sensing, feeling, and thinking all involved not just your mind but your heart as well. Thus the character for "thinking" and the one for "sensing and feeling" both contain the heart-mind radical. The ancients believed that we did our sensing, feeling, and thinking with only one organ.

In the last twenty years, cognitive science and neuroscience have finally caught up with the ancients and "proven" the unity of mind and body. Having finally discarded the reductionistic paradigm, they now know that the mind's ability to refine movement by coordinating some 630 muscles with greater precision—a process otherwise known as learning—is inextricably linked to the body's ability to sense and feel. After three centuries, Western science has returned to the age-old concept that the mind is something much deeper and all-encompassing than cold synapses firing between your ears.

As we shall see in the following chapters, your mind has the potential to sense and feel at extraordinarily subtle levels and in the process direct your movement with the precision of an Olympic athlete, concert pianist, or Bagua master. Each of us can choose to move toward that potential or away from it by either developing or suppressing our sensibility—that is, our *sense-ability*. When we suppress our sense-ability, we begin to lose just that: our ability to accurately sense and feel. In the process, we sacrifice not only coordination, strength, balance, and agility, but something even more fundamental.

The less we choose to sense and feel on our own, the more we must rely on external sources to do the sensing and feeling for us. Put another way, the less precisely we can direct ourselves, the more we end up relying on someone else to do the directing for us. We may, for example, rely on a heart-rate monitor to tell us how hard and long to exercise. We may trust calorie counters to tell us how much to eat. We may rely on fashion magazines to tell us how to look. And we may look to running experts to tell us how to run.

Yet, each of us has the potential to leapfrog past experts and other external sources if we only pay attention to what is deep down inside of us— that is, if we start cultivating, rather than suppressing, our sense-abilities. When you cultivate your sense-ability, you are in effect connecting with your heart and thereby cultivating your mind. And a sense-able mind is not only the best, but moreover the only instrument capable of guiding you toward your vast potential. There are no substitutes. The more you dull your sense-abilities, the more you blunt the very instrument designed to lead you toward improvement.

How Did We Lose Our Senses?

What we call upbringing or education is a way of making children conform to the conventions of society.... In the process, most children are—perhaps unavoidably—warped. They lose their innocence and their spontaneity, their unselfconsciousness. In psychological jargon, they possess all kinds of inner conflicts and complexities, and they do not seem to be able to recover from them in adult life without the expense of psychoanalysis or some similar kind of therapy. And even then, I am not quite sure how often they really recover.

—ALAN WATTS

Losing our senses begins early in life because doing so allows us to get along. To one degree or another we must comply with parents, teachers, bosses—in short, authority, in order to make it through childhood, school, and later, the working world. Think about this: what typically happens to children when they don't obey their parents and teachers? What happens to adults when they don't obey their bosses? What happens if you don't file your income taxes?

This is not to say that everybody always bows to authority. Sometimes we exhibit a healthy disregard for people, organizations, or even ideological constraints that may be squelching our inner sanctum. We may, for example, leave a school, job, or even profession that does not suit us. Mostly, however, we are playing a survival game called "fitting in." Whether we are trying to be in with the "in" crowd or the "out" crowd doesn't matter. The simple fact that we are trying to be something means trying not to be something else. It means turning off our senses to some degree and suppressing essential parts of ourselves.

Fitting in is not, in and of itself, intrinsically bad. Without some compliance to those around us, we would have no culture, and arguably, no human race. Too much compliance, however, and we end up with a society of automatons, with no connection to the beating of their own heart.

Look at the clothes you're wearing, the kind of haircut you're sporting, and the things hanging on the wall in your home and you instantly know to which club you either belong or are trying to belong. Perhaps more striking, notice when something inside you reacts to the way another person is dressed. That something inside is saying, "I'm definitely not in that club." Each club, whether the British Royal Family, Hell's Angels, or the "I don't belong to any club" club has characteristic codes of behavior—or in other words, characteristic codes of moving. The question is how well do the movement dictates of your club really suit your individual desires and needs? How much does moving the "right" way mean cutting yourself off from your own senses? How much have you distanced yourself from the beating of your own heart?

Compliance taken too far means moving in a way that is not in accord with who you are. And when you are not in accord with who you are, you are literally uncomfortable, because while your body desires to move one way, you are forcing it to move another. You are busy trying to be what you are not, and this contradiction can be literally felt in your body. Yet because your body does not stop talking, the only way to live with this contradiction is to ignore the language of your body, namely sensing and feeling. Living in contradiction means, in short, disabling your sense-ability.

Have You Lost Your Mind?

Within an authoritarian atmosphere ... repetitions carry seeds of corruption. The practice necessary for skill is done in a context that rewards conformity to someone else's ideas rather than finding one's own way. The infant is permitted its brief moment of trial and error before learning that there are right and wrong ways of doing things. Doing things "right" becomes more important than learning.

—DON HANLON JOHNSON,
*BODY: RECOVERING OUR
SENSUAL WISDOM*

As I mentioned earlier, your magnificent measuring instrument, capable of feeling and sensing to extraordinary levels of subtlety, doesn't just reside in the gray matter between your ears. It actually encompasses your entire body. It exists in your left little toe, and in your right elbow; in your liver and in your large intestine; in your blood vessels and in your lymph nodes. Because sensing and feeling occur throughout your body, your mind lives everywhere in it. This is why some people refer to the body and mind as the "bodymind."[1]

It follows that when you begin to lose your senses, you also begin to lose your mind, which doesn't mean you are going insane. It simply means that you are not in touch with your own sense-abilities. Since sanity is defined by

---

[1] Ken Dychtwald has authored a pioneering book on the subject, aptly titled *Bodymind* (New York: Pantheon, 1977).

how the majority of people behave in society, you could say that losing your mind has actually become the norm—our cultural standard, in other words, of sanity. This being the case, people who maintain their sense-abilities and therefore don't lose their minds are ironically considered at least a little insane.[2]

Not surprisingly, our "sane" culture, which encourages and sometimes even enforces the muting of our sense-abilities, exacts a heavy price from its inhabitants in the form of deadening our innate curiosity and aliveness, inhibiting learning and improvement, and actually encouraging self-destructive tendencies. Our "sane" culture, in other words, encourages a great deal of mindless behavior.

How does this happen?

Just as muscles begin to atrophy when you don't use them, senses begin to dull when you ignore them. Since losing your sense-ability means losing your ability to distinguish between what feels good and what doesn't, it also means losing your ability to distinguish between what is good for you and what isn't.

Nature has equipped all living creatures with the ability to distinguish between what feels good and what doesn't in order to give all forms of life the maximum chance for survival. Without this ability, they begin to self-destruct, and not just in the figurative sense. People who lack ability to feel pain, for example—such as those suffering from Hansen's disease—will unwittingly cause so much damage to themselves that they eventually become disfigured. NFL football players perform a similar task when they are given painkillers or smelling salts for serious injuries and are then sent back on the field (Here, it is not only considered sane but heroic to sacrifice your body in an effort to win). Until recently, the media reported so little on the condition in which these athletes found themselves after leaving the gridiron that most of the public mistakenly believed they led normal lives.

---

[2] Given this, it should be no surprise that those who forge deeper connections with their senses are often thought to be at least a little crazy, even though they form the ranks of every society's innovators and pioneers.

For the rest of us who aren't in the NFL or suffering from Hansen's disease, we nonetheless play similar, albeit less dramatic, roles in hurting ourselves. How could we not when we have lost our senses?

While just about everybody understands the feeling of acute pain, many of us have lost the ability to clearly distinguish between other sensations—namely ones that do not register as acute pain. Many of us, in other words, tend not to notice lesser discomforts that nonetheless impinge on the quality of our movement, mood, and well-being. On the surface, it may sound like a good thing to be able to ignore pain and discomfort—if only to save money on doctor's bills and trips to the drugstore. But as I mentioned above, feeling pain and even minor discomfort is a necessary tool by which humans, and indeed, all living creatures keep from destroying themselves.

Whereas acute pain normally signals sudden trauma, subtler discomforts signal damage that is either imminent or in the process of occurring, albeit at a slower pace. So when we ignore minor discomfort, we are ignoring something that is either potentially or actively destructive.

Yin and Yang: Why Pain Is Important

If I am well practiced at blocking out as much pain as possible, I may eventually lose my ability to distinguish between subtleties of discomfort—and just as importantly, subtleties of comfort. If I continue to push myself to extremes of pain tolerance, I may reach a point where anything short of acute pain no longer registers. In such cases I will still be able to tell the difference between pulling a hamstring and not pulling a hamstring, or throwing out my back and not throwing it out, but gross distinctions are not enough to move, and therefore live, the way I want to. All the distinctions that give me greater self-awareness and thereby provide me with more power, agility, coordination, and gracefulness will have been lost. What I will be missing, in other words, are not only the messengers alerting me of acute injury, but the extraordinarily rich and varied world of distinctions that lies between acute pain and its absence.

In our fast-paced, results-driven, "no pain, no gain" society, it is not only our ability to feel pain that we relinquish, but our ability to feel at all. And this means that by diminishing our ability to feel pain, we also diminish our ability to feel pleasure.

Chinese philosophers of antiquity divided the world into a duality of yin and yang—opposing phenomena that depend on each other to exist. Because yin and yang are mutually dependent halves necessary to create the whole of human experience, neither was considered to be good or bad. To have light, you must have dark. Hot exists only because there is cold. As I mentioned earlier, to have a mind, you must have a body. And pleasure exists because of pain. You cannot extinguish one without extinguishing the other.

I believe this is one of the reasons so few people enjoy running. Instead of taking heed of pain, they try to suppress it. And in doing so, they minimize the possibility of feeling pleasure.

Here's how it works.

If I force myself to run regularly even though I don't like running, it's probably because I don't derive much pleasure from the activity. What I will clearly notice is the discomfort that comes from running—perhaps the burning of muscles, the fatigue, the tedium, and maybe even the tweaking of parts of my body to which I am unwittingly causing injury. If I continue to plow my way through the discomfort, relying on willpower to carry me through, then I am not paying heed to my discomfort. I am probably blocking it out—perhaps even listening to music at the same time so as to distract myself from the pain. Each time I will my way through this process, I am ignoring the voices inside me saying things like, "this is unpleasant," "I really don't want to be doing this," or "this hurts." Obviously, I am not increasing my discomfort (at least not until I finally incur a major injury), but I am also not increasing the pleasure I could be experiencing in the process.

What if, on other hand, I started listening to my senses and feelings? I might then want to slow down. Initially I might not run as far. I might start my run by walking. I might even notice how I was rolling off my right foot and how that differed from how I rolled off my left foot. When I felt discomfort, I would likely change what I was doing, experimenting

with ways that could not only make me feel better, but grant me the pleasure of finding things out (to borrow an oft-quoted phrase from Richard
Feynman).[3]

In the process of listening, I would start to know who I am and be able
to compare it to who I was trying to be—someone in a hurry to get the run
over with. I would begin to understand how I was running, and that awareness alone could help to guide me toward a better way of running. The act
of feeling and sensing myself instantaneously creates new neural pathways,
and this means new movement possibilities. While it is likely that I might
go slower at times, run fewer miles, and even revert to walking from time to
time, it is also more likely that I would discover how to run faster and with
more pleasure. And if running started giving me more pleasure, I would
likely end up running more than I did when I wasn't paying attention to my
feelings—not that getting yourself to run more should be your goal.

Let's compare your average runner to your average child running around
on the playground. The average runner slogs her way through at a steady pace
and often a grimace on her face. The average child on the playground varies her
pace—sometimes sprinting, sometimes walking, sometimes darting, sometimes leaping, sometimes lying down, and sometimes squealing with delight.
Which one seems to have more energy? Who ends up running farther?

If you watch children (particularly those who haven't been introduced
to video games), their energy seems boundless. They could run around on
the playground for hours without tiring. We, on the other hand, often feel
tired even before we take our first step. I believe this is because children pay
attention to discomfort. They either avoid it or find ways to mitigate it. They
also pay attention to pleasure and actually seek it out. They walk when they
want to walk, and sprint when they want to sprint. In fact, it is in slowing

---

[3] Asked for his thoughts about winning the Nobel Prize, Feynman replied: "I don't see
that it makes any point that someone in the Swedish Academy decides that this work
is noble enough to receive a prize—I've already got the prize. The prize is the pleasure
of finding the thing out, the kick in the discovery, the observation that other people
use [my work]—those are the real things, the honors are unreal to me." Richard P.
Feynman quoted in Jeffrey Robbins, ed., *The Pleasure of Finding Things Out: The Best
Short Works of Richard P. Feynman* (New York: Perseus, 1999), 12.

down and walking that they gain the desire to run and sprint—not because they are in a hurry, but because the human mind likes variation. Running is a wonderful variant to walking. It is the yang to the yin of walking.

I have played enough basketball, tennis, and soccer to know that people inherently like to run. But they like it only when it brings them pleasure. You will find that many of the fittest basketball, tennis, and soccer players don't like running, even though during a game or match, they actually run more than most runners. All they need is a ball to chase and they're off to the races. By chasing a ball, they are chasing their pleasure. And as a runner, this is what you could be doing: following your pleasure.

CHASING WAVES

A game I like to play when I go to the ocean is something I call "chasing waves." As the tide goes out, I shuffle as a boxer would toward the receding water. As a wave starts crashing toward the shore, I wait until the last minute and then shuffle or simply run as fast as I can away from the water. Depending on how large the wave is, I give myself more or less distance from its shoreward crashing.

A nice element of this game is that there is so much possibility built into it. Depending on both the time of day, month, and year, the tide will be closer to shore or farther out, the waves consequently rolling in faster or slower. This means that along with the variation in speed, I'm dealing with a variation in grade because the slope on which I'm chasing and being chased is either flatter (when the tide is lower) or steeper (when the tide is higher). It also means that the sand on which I'm running is either firmer or looser.

On top of all of the environmental variation, I get to choose any number of ways to chase and be chased, often becoming thoroughly engrossed as I imagine a child would be, and all the while enjoying the sunshine, fresh air, and ocean water. Meanwhile, in my enjoyment, I am inadvertently strengthening my body—particularly since my toes, ankles, and metatarsals get to move in ways they normally wouldn't when encased in shoes and walking on concrete.

7

To Be or Not to Be

I hate tennis, hate it with all my heart, and I keep playing, keep hit-ting all morning, all afternoon because I have no choice. No matter how much I want to stop, I don't. I keep begging myself to stop, and I keep playing, and this gap, this contradiction between what I want to do and what I actually do feels like the core of my life.

—ANDRE AGASSI, *OPEN: AN AUTOBIOGRAPHY*

Seventh grade marked the end of my days of playing and exploring when overnight, boys my age seemed to have grown to twice my size and gained the power and speed to match. In an attempt to catch up with them, I began to abide by the principle of always pushing my limits. Looking back, it isn't surprising that by the time ninth grade rolled around I had already associated running with a great deal of pain and misery. Regardless of the fact that at one point I was winning junior varsity races, there was little joy to be had in either training or competing. And while it is true that I enjoyed a sudden spike in popularity during the brief time I was winning, the act of running itself remained, for me, mostly drudgery. Later, when the friends and attention disappeared—they tend to evaporate when your competition improves and you start coming in tenth place—I had to summon more willpower to continue.

By tenth grade, I was becoming increasingly unenthusiastic about lifting my head off the pillow when my alarm went off. On designated "hard," days when I knew our coach would be squeezing every last ounce of juice from our legs, I became sullen and irritable. At this point I was running with the varsity squad, and as its slowest member, barely able to keep up. The build-up to races was even worse. Though it seems preposterous in retrospect, I distinctly remember warming up before many races with a sudden empathy for everyone who had ever been sent to the gallows.

School itself was simply another version of running in that those who struggled were simply encouraged to try harder. The problem, however, was not one of insufficient effort. With my short attention span and propensity to get caught up in the tiniest details, I would often find myself reading the same paragraph over and over. Each day felt like I was falling farther behind.

Exhausted from running and unable to concentrate, I spent countless nights battling a desire to either catch a snippet of television or a snack from the cupboard. Nine o'clock and still unable to figure out my first math problem, I would eat a bagel. Ten o'clock and I'd switch to physics:

Centripetal force is a force that makes a body follow a curved path: it is always directed orthogonal to the velocity of the body, toward the instantaneous center of curvature of the path.

Huh? Time to order a pizza. Two hours and a painfully bloated stomach later, my books continued to stare back impassively. If I was learning anything, it was how not to learn.

In the classroom things seemed equally complex. I often slept through chemistry and math, while in English my fear of looking stupid kept me on red alert and praying that the teacher wouldn't call my name. My classmates seemed impossibly smart as they rolled off expert, polysyllabic opinions on the three-hundred-page Victorian novel we were supposed to have finished. In the two weeks we were given to read it, two dozen bagels, three pizzas, and one trip to the gastroenterologist couldn't get me past page 22.

Obviously, trying harder wasn't working. Little did I know in high school, both learning and running can be joyful. By fixating too heavily on results, however—be it the "right" answer, the good grade, or the faster time—I had taken the process out of the process, and thus, the learning out of the learning.

Each day in cross-country, for example, I would go to practice expecting to be in over my head. All the tension, anxiety, and defeat revealed themselves not only in the grim expression I carried through most of the day but in my posture, which was a combination of over-tightness in certain areas and collapse in others. I had become an unwitting participant in my own oppression, piling sandbags on my own shoulders. My attitude, in other words, created a whole neuromuscular response that actually made my body feel heavier and my mind duller. Rather than living life, I was surviving it.

"Why did you continue on this way?" one might ask. "No sensible person would do this to himself."

This is indeed true: no sense-able person would treat himself this way.

Being Versus Trying to Be (Productive)

We have become a civilization based on work—not even "productive work" but work as an end and meaning in itself. We have come to believe that men and women who do not work harder than they wish at jobs they do not particularly enjoy are bad people unworthy of love, care, or assistance from their communities. It is as if we have collectively acquiesced to our own enslavement.

—DAVID GRAEBER, *BULLSHIT JOBS: A THEORY*

You may have noticed that the vast majority of practicing, training, and working is more about getting the job done than how it gets done, more about getting results than learning. For most people, practice means focusing on the ends while letting the means slip far off into the background. In this manner, practice often becomes more about trying to force the ends rather than allowing them to occur naturally.

Obviously, getting the job done, getting results, or in other words, being productive is important. Productivity is how skyscrapers, homes, and cars get built. It is what allows us to put food on the table. Productivity is vital because it provides not only some measure of accomplishment, but at its core, some means for surviving.[1]

Yet, what if there is more to life than surviving?[2]

If I take a step back and ask not just what I am practicing, but how I am practicing what I am practicing, I begin to discover who I am being when I am doing what I am doing. And who I am being when I am doing what I am doing will affect the outcome of what I am doing. This is because being is shorthand for both being present and being myself.

Being present means being completely tuned in to what I am sensing and feeling. If as we saw earlier, sensing and feeling determines the quality of my movement, being present, which heightens my sensing and feeling, then enriches the quality of my movement.

As we shall see below, being myself is the act of knowing myself through sensing and feeling myself. So, if I am being present and therefore completely tuned in to my sensing and feeling, then I am also being myself at the same time. To be present, in other words, is to be myself.

Trying to Be Could Put You at the Bottom of the Ocean

Good runners get from A to B faster than average runners because they pay attention to their senses and feelings and consequently drop any parasitic tension that would otherwise get in their way. In other words, they improve the quality of their movement by sensing and feeling more, and in this manner devote their efforts to being, rather than trying to be, good runners.

---

[1] Though one could argue that productivity is about making profits, it is important to understand that in our current political economy, profits are crucial to the survival of any entity, from the smallest one-person operation to the largest multinational conglomerates.

[2] By this statement I do not mean to denigrate anyone living under difficult conditions. A refugee, an undocumented worker, or even a single parent working at Walmart obviously has far fewer choices than, say, a typical member of the professional class. The fact that in the world's wealthiest nation alone, tens of millions are so limited in their choices that they are essentially consigned to live years, if not their entire lives, struggling to survive obviously says more about the kind of world we live in than it does the individual.

Average runners, on the other hand, try to be better. But trying to be presupposes that being isn't good enough. It is the negation of being in the belief that not being is somehow better. For example, if I say, "I am trying to be a better runner," this means that who I am is not good enough. But this is based on the assumption that I know who I am. And as we shall see shortly, most of us don't, holding instead a grossly inaccurate approximation of who we are. In other words, we think we know who we are when we really don't, the result of which is that in trying not to be who we think we are, we end up trying not to be who we are not. All of this may sound confusing, but perhaps the following analogy will help your understanding.

If I want to get to Chicago and I am in New York, it makes sense to drive west in order to get there. If I want to get to Chicago and think I'm in New York when I'm really in San Francisco, driving west will appear to make sense, but doing so will put me at the bottom of the Pacific Ocean. The upshot here is, if I want to get to Chicago, it is important to know who I am—in this particular case, a person in San Francisco, not a person in New York.

Knowing Means Feeling

You can't do what you want if you don't know what you're doing.

—MOSHE FELDENKRAIS

Frequently repeated by Feldenkrais teachers, the preceding quote is really another way of saying, "You can't do what you want if you don't sense what you're doing." This is because knowing and sensing are actually one and the same phenomenon. Thus, the more you sense yourself, the more you know yourself. Conversely, the less you sense yourself, the less you know yourself. And the less you know yourself, the more you're like the person in San Francisco who tries to get to Chicago by driving West.

We can shorten all of this by simply saying, if you don't sense what you're doing, then you are busy not being, rather than being, yourself. And when you're busy not being rather than being, you can't do what you want.

If you understand this principle, then you will understand that the key to running with more power is not to try to run like an Olympian, but rather to run like yourself. And the funny thing is, the more you run like yourself rather than trying to run like an Olympian, the more you will actually run like an Olympian. (Yes, you read the last sentence correctly.)

It's really that simple. Yet at the same time, it is difficult. We have spent so many years taking the hard way that we often know no other way. Making life difficult has become a habit.

Common Non-sense

To run like yourself, you have to know how you are actually running. And to discover how you are running, you have to sense and feel what you are doing when you run. Unfortunately, we live in a culture whose version of common sense encourages us to block out our senses. Our senses are, in this manner, becoming *non*-senses. From the standpoint of improving and learning, it makes no sense—or perhaps more aptly put, non-sense—to mute your sense-abilities when doing so decreases power, speed, coordination, and agility while dramatically increasing your chances of hurting yourself.

As stated in the previous two chapters, improving your sense-ability leads to reducing internal conflict, thereby increasing your control over the 630 muscles in your body. What's more, if you consider that muting your sense-ability simultaneously decreases your ability to know what is good for you and what isn't, then doing so also increases your reliance on others to tell you what is good for you. And if you are relying on others to decide what is good for you, then you are giving up your responsibility—that is, response-*ability*. When you sense less, in other words, you not only give up control over your own body but your ability to respond appropriately to your own desires and needs. Sensing less you become less response-*able*.

Because sensing and feeling are inextricably tied to emotions, suppressing feelings can have similar effects on both your sense-ability and response-ability. Emotions, as we will see in chapter 9, "Who Turned Up the Gravity?," play a pivotal role in movement. When you try not to be sad, angry, or in pain by suppressing your feelings of sadness, anger, or pain, you are effectively stifling both your movement possibilities and response-ability in one fell swoop. Of course, doing so may be helpful in temporarily allowing you to fit in better (read, not show "negative" emotions, or in some cases, any emotions at all), deal with physical trauma, or simply make it through your workday, but habitual not being—that is, habitual suppressing of your sensing and feeling—comes at a cost.

Even without the use of drugs, many of us have already become habituated not to feel and therefore not to know ourselves. And we have spent so much time not feeling that we have actually lost much of the sensation in our own bodies. I experienced this firsthand after years of forcing myself to do things that I didn't like to do, such as continue running. And as my sense-ability decreased, so did my coordination, power, and speed. The frightening part about all of this was that I had become so accustomed to being numb that I unconsciously regarded my anaesthetized way of living as normal (even though I consciously felt miserable).

Once again, I am not alone.

A culture that places a premium on hurrying about, enduring discomfort at all costs, and thereby "getting it done" is a culture that anaesthetizes its inhabitants. Not only have many physical ailments such as knee, back, neck, and shoulder problems become the norm, but so have grim faces, forced smiles, and perfunctory greetings. We as an entire culture have become so accustomed to not feeling, not knowing, and not being that these abnormal ways of living are now regarded as normal.

~~What's~~ Who's Stopping You?

I have taught many children and teenagers who were caught up in the belief that their self-worth depended on how well they performed at tennis and other skills.... Children who have been taught to measure themselves in this way often become adults driven by a compulsion to succeed, which overshadows all else. The tragedy of this belief is not that they will fail to find the success they seek, but that they will not discover the love or even the self-respect they were led to believe will come with it.

—W. TIMOTHY GALLWEY, *THE INNER GAME OF TENNIS*

Trying to be and the consequent loss of sense-ability is, in short, a difficult way to live—or perhaps more aptly put, not quite live—because it means engaging in an internal battle. Trying to be something that I'm not, which is equivalent to trying not to feel who I am, is essentially like a game of football where I am playing defense against myself. This means that I am diverting a great deal of energy toward defeating myself the way the defense attempts to defeat the opposing offense. At the same time, I am trying my hardest to score a touch-down, meaning I am trying to succeed. Trying to be thus translates to all of the work it takes to both score a touchdown and at the same time stop myself from scoring a touchdown. It requires the work of running an offense, and at the same time, running a defense that is trying to defeat the offense.

What do you think the outcome is? Watch a professional football game sometime and you will see tempers flaring, bodies colliding, voices straining, and nerves on edge. This is how many of us are unwittingly not quite living our lives. The conflicts and collisions may be internal and therefore remain somewhat hidden, but their evidence is betrayed by a host of physical and emotional disorders such as headaches, backaches, arthritis, insomnia, fibro-myalgia, and depression, to name a few.

Many see such problems as an inevitable part of living in our fast-paced world. Many ailments are even considered to be part and parcel of the mys-terious phenomenon medical experts call "aging." Yet if a culture drives people toward such suffering, what does it say about that culture?

For those of you who suffer, consider that on some level, dysfunction in a dysfunctional society (like ours) could be normal—even if specialists want to give you a drug for it. In a culture of common non-sense, in other words, dysfunction is like a big flashing billboard on the freeway of life saying, "Look here! There is another way!"

If Trying Harder Didn't Work ...

If trying hard didn't work, trying harder is doing more of what didn't work.

—CHARLES EISENSTEIN

Trying to be, which could simply be another way of saying, trying harder without necessarily knowing who I am being or how I am doing what I am doing, normally translates to doing more of what I was doing before. So if like most people I am already playing defense on myself, trying harder means revving up the offense and defense at the same time. It is like stepping harder on the gas pedal when my engine is already overheating. Looking at it this way, the harder I try, the smaller my returns per measure of effort.

This is why, for most people, there is an element of strain accompanying their increases in effort. Strain can be read as an excessive amount of muscle contraction that not only contributes nothing to moving you forward but actually contributes something to slowing you down by pulling in undesired directions. Those directions could be down, up, sideways, and even backward. This means that for everyone, including Olympic runners, trying harder can actually result in increasing the amount of force pulling in the wrong directions.

The difficulties don't end there, because as I mentioned earlier, misdirected force does not simply disappear. Some of it inevitably ends up getting stuck in your joints, causing excessive compression, torsion, or shearing stress (shearing force is what causes a coffee mug to slide off the kitchen table during an earthquake)—one reason why people who run with less power and ease also tend to get injured more easily.

In sharp contrast to trying to be, being remains the deepest part of us that only fully emerges after we remove all of the superimposed ideas that had been stacked on top. Instead of remaining shackled by thoughts about who we should be—often leading us to try to be who we are not—being allows us to come to our senses and draw forth what simply is. No longer playing defense on our self, something new then begins to flow through our body and mind.

The Bagua and Taichi masters refer to this flow as qi (sometimes written as chi). They spend years unblocking and channeling it by tuning in to different sensations in their bodies. This tuning-in is the refinement of intention. As their intention becomes more and more refined, freeing them of unintended, parasitic contractions, their movement becomes more and more fluid and powerful.

From a biomechanical point of view, being allows force that was previously blocked or misdirected—resulting in less coordination and power—to travel unimpeded through your skeleton, resulting in more coordination and power. Being, in other words, allows for a much smoother translation of force, thereby giving you far greater power and precision in movement. This smooth translation is how Bagua masters effortlessly toss people twice their weight through the air, and how good runners propel themselves swiftly and smoothly to the finish line.

When you engage your sense-abilities, you not only generate more power, but you stimulate the flow of everything from cerebral spinal fluid to oxygen, blood and lymph, and other bodily liquids, gases, and solids. Like unblocking a dam inside your own body, muscles that were previously tense begin to release themselves and their constriction on all the vessels, tissues, and organs beneath them, thereby freeing the nutrients and waste materials that were previously trapped within each to be easily transported.

In addition to increasing the flow of liquids, gases, and solids, being changes the flow of electrochemicals through your nervous system. By letting go of parasitic contractions, you sidestep the old well-worn neural pathways associated with constriction in order to generate new neural pathways—those associated with freedom of movement. Loosening the muscular straightjacket actually frees up your nervous system to create new, more sense-able pathways, such as those that awaken dormant muscles and tendons to direct force to where you want it to go.

When you begin to understand that being nurtures the flow of everything from mechanical force to blood, lymph, and electrochemicals, you can more easily see that being is simply life itself coursing through your entire body. Thus, the more you are being, the more you embody life. Conversely, the less you are being—or in other words, the more you are trying to be— the more you hinder the flow of life.

Running Versus Shuffling

As a final note on being, I recommend you tune into your level of pleasure every time you go for a run. If you begin noticing a consistent lack of enthusiasm, it means that part of you does not want to be running. And, as elucidated in chapter 5, "Intention," the internal conflict will play out as parasitic contractions in some parts of yourself and a simultaneous collapse in others. The most obvious example of such conflict is when you see people shuffling through their daily "run." Shuffling is not running. Only running is running, and it is important not to confuse the two. The more you shuffle and call it running, the more you not only habituate your body to moving in highly limited ranges of motion, but also convince your mind into accepting this misrepresentation as running. By conflating shuffling and running, in other words, you are not only teaching yourself to move with restriction, but allowing a half-hearted imitation of running to stand for the real thing. Furthermore, the internal conflict and consequent increase in strain means that you are unconsciously linking the idea of running with struggle and displeasure, rather than freedom and pleasure.

If you set out to run and end up shuffling for a good portion of the time, I recommend calling what you have done a "shuffle" instead of a "run." It is important to have an accurate label, and at the same time let go of any judgment you might have on that label because, as with anything else, shuffling is neither intrinsically good nor bad, as long as you are aware that you are doing it. If done with awareness and clear intention, shuffling can even be a tool to improve your running, which is why I have devoted Lessons 18 and 19 to exploring the action.

By making a clear distinction between running and shuffling, you are clarifying your intention so that when your intention is to run, you really do run, even if only for half a block. Conversely, when you need to stop and rest, you won't find yourself shuffling out of a compulsion to keep working, even though your body is telling you to do otherwise. By keeping your intention clear, you will be fully invested in running when you are running and fully resting when you are resting. Meanwhile, you will be stepping away from the conflicted netherworld of half-running, half-resting, or otherwise going through the motions. As a result, not only will your running stand a better chance of improving, but you will become more in tune with your own body, allowing it to rest when it truly wants to rest and exert itself when it truly wants to exert itself. Along with this, you will get far more enjoyment out of the process of either shuffling or running because you will be more aware of what you are really doing, which will in turn allow you to more accurately do what you really want to do. Once again, we come back to Moshe Feldenkrais's insightful statement, "You can't do what you want if you don't know what you're doing."

The next time you notice yourself shuffling when your intention was to run, take pause. Perhaps you are simply too tired to continue running. Perhaps shuffling has become a habit, and you've lost touch with the joy of running. In either case I recommend you stop and walk rather than shuffle. Otherwise, by shuffling without intending to shuffle, you are actually showing your nervous system how not to run, and more importantly, you are habituating yourself to not being. This is why running enthusiastically for a hundred meters and then stopping is far more beneficial to learning and improving than shuffling for ten miles when you'd rather be doing something else.

Finally, if you are having difficulty getting motivated to run, I recommend you not force yourself. Skip to chapter 15, "Compulsion," if you want to read more on how forcing can undermine motivation. Check out the experiment at the end of the chapter, titled "Running For the Pleasure of It," if you are seeking an alternative to auto-authoritarianism. Whatever you do, keep in mind that millions of people around the world do not run and are perfectly happy, healthy, and in shape.

PART 2   PRACTICAL MATTERS

8

Imitation: Why Trying to Run Like an Olympian Keeps You from Running Like an Olympian

If you stop a hundred people at random and ask them to evaluate their driving ability, every single one will say, "above average." It is a scientific fact that all drivers, including those who are going the wrong way on interstate highways, believe they are above average. Not me, of course. I am currently ranked fourth among the top drivers in world history, between Mario Andretti and Spartacus.

—DAVE BARRY

Several summers ago I returned to Tianjin after spending an entire fall, winter, and spring training rigorously on my own. It had been almost a year since I had seen the masters, so I had a lot to show them. Eager to impress, I arrived early to greet Master Li on the first day of training. A diminutive man lacking the girth and bravado of Master Ge, Master Li nonetheless carried an air of quiet self-assurance. Judging by his size and reticence, you wouldn't suspect that he had defeated high-level challengers from all over the city. Yet, once you saw him in action, or perhaps more accurately, lost sight of him in action, you knew you were in the hands of someone special. Master Li had a special knack of disappearing when going over two-person drills. One moment he was in front of you, and the next he was behind you or at your flank. Meanwhile, his iron hands always came from nowhere, usually stopping half-an-inch from your face or some vital point on your body.

"Show me the first form," Master Li commanded, in his usual quiet but stern manner.

I began. Within seconds I heard him muttering something below his breath. Then a clear, "Stop." Master Li looked vaguely disinterested, as if he had better things to do. I hesitated.

"Stop," he repeated, sensing my desire to continue. "Show me the second form."

Ten seconds into the second form, and again, unintelligible muttering. "Stop," he said, with a hint of irritation. Master Li was apparently not nearly as impressed as I was.

"Third form," he said under his breath, as if ordering from a menu. He was looking at his watch.

I was hesitant to even begin. Obviously we should just call it off and go have breakfast. Ten seconds into the third form and I already knew what was coming.

This time there was no continuing. Master Li began to rattle off everything that I had been doing wrong. He pointed out places where he said I was rushing and not paying attention—places, in other words, where I lacked awareness. Quite a lot of "wrongness," considering my performance lasted a total of thirty seconds. I meanwhile stood in disbelief, feeling more than a little defiant knowing that it couldn't be as bad as he made it out to be.

Later, when I returned to my dormitory, I decided to film myself going over the beginning of each form. Upon seeing myself in the viewfinder, I immediately knew that Master Li was right on all points. There were indeed many flaws in my form, even if I had improved since the previous year. Obviously, I had not been fully aware of how I had been moving. And until Master Li pointed out my mistakes, and they were corroborated by the camera, I was unaware that I was unaware.

Know Thyself: The Three Cardinal Questions

In order to do what someone else is doing, you must first know what you yourself are doing. If you don't, then you'll be like the person in San Francisco who tries to get to Chicago by driving west.

The knowing I'm referring to is actually not a static state but a process of discovery and creation. If we pare it down to simple body mechanics, knowing yourself means discovering how you use the ground to generate force, how you translate this force through your body, and how new neural pathways are created in the entire process. If the ground is a springboard, your muscles are what direct the spring from the springboard through your body when you take off, and they are what directs the spring from your body back into the springboard when you land. Consequently, any lack of spring when you take off and any excessive *thud* when you land will be due to your muscles misdirecting the force.

All of this may sound complicated, but it really isn't if we view the concept of "know thyself" as a matter of understanding how to more efficiently direct our take-off and landing. It boils down to what I call the Three Cardinal Questions:

How much effort does it take to move from one position to the next (and therefore, how can I minimize the effort)?

How solid is my connection with the ground?

Does it feel good?

Number one: How much effort does it take to move from one position to the next?

The less effort it takes to perform a given task—whether lifting a finger or running the hundred-meter dash—the less extraneous tension I will carry in my body, and the lighter and more powerful I will feel.

Number two: How clear is my connection with the ground?

Whether I am sitting, standing, walking, or even lying down, my connection with the ground will reveal two important things: (1) How much extraneous tension I am carrying in my body, and (2) How much I'm collapsing in places where muscles are not fully supporting my structure.

The more tension I carry, the more that parts of me will unnecessarily pull away from the floor, making my contact with the floor less clear, precise, and solid. This sort of tension could be reflected anywhere in my body—for example, in a tightness in my belly, a clenching in my jaw, a rising of my shoulders—and all of it serves to divert my center of gravity, pull me off balance, and thereby affect how my feet or any other part (if I am sitting or lying down) make contact with the floor. Rather than feeling grounded into the floor, I will feel off-balance and out of kilter. Rather than pushing off with power and precision, my stepping will feel murky and unclear, perhaps akin to sloshing through mud.

While some muscles exhibit parasitic tension, others will likely remain chronically underused and relatively dormant. This further exacerbates the problem because the dormant muscles are not being used to do what they are designed for—namely, counterbalancing muscles that pull a particular joint in the opposite direction. The predictable result is further imbalance and less precision in how I make contact with the floor. Parts of my feet, for example, may collapse into the floor—the extreme example being fallen arches. And as we saw in chapter 5, "Intention," a collapse in any part of my body will affect the way that I use my entire body.

Number three: Does it feel good?

Pleasure and pain are the two most potent forces that guide movement and behavior. If it doesn't feel good, then it probably isn't good for me. By finding ways to feel good, I actually transform my ways of moving, and therefore, my ways of being in the world. One way to look at it is that the fastest, most powerful ways to run are also the most pleasurable ways to run.

Distinctions

What asking the Three Cardinal Questions brings to light is who you are beneath the (superimposed) parasitic contractions. By wondering, in other words, you begin to shed unnecessary holdings associated with trying to be. This means as you ask, you shall be given—in this case a whole new world of distinction, discovery, and transformation.

Making distinctions is in and of itself transformational because the human nervous system is actually wired with feedback loops in such a way that new neural pathways are created every time you discover with greater precision what it is that you are doing. These new pathways then become part of a new way of directing your muscles and therefore a new way of moving. And since movement is all that defines human behavior and expression, we can accurately say that making such distinctions results in a new way of being. In the process of making distinctions and thereby knowing yourself, you are actually transforming yourself without trying to transform yourself.

From a practical standpoint, making distinctions results in greater precision in movement which can fundamentally improve the mechanics of your stride. To test the veracity of the last sentence, get ready to do Lesson 12, "Mobilizing Your Rib Cage." If you explore the lesson slowly and attentively, you will actually improve your mechanical efficiency because you will be making the distinction between your unconscious habit of having your foot on the brakes, so to speak, and the new conscious act of taking it off. Making the distinction is in and of itself what takes your foot off the brakes and therefore what allows you to generate more power, since effort that was previously devoted to slowing you down can now be used to speed you up.

Not surprisingly, Bagua masters are champions of making distinctions. To make finer distinctions, they break movements down into smaller pieces, slow down, and pay very close attention to what they are sensing and feeling. To stop slowing themselves down unintentionally, they first do it intentionally.

Making distinctions is, in fact, how all humans sift out parasitic muscle tension and consequently gain more control and thus more precision, power, and coordination. Without the ability to make distinctions, we would have no possibility of improving the precision, power, and coordination with which we move. In fact, we would have no precision, power, and coordination at all.

Each time you make a new distinction, new neural pathways get formed in your brain. The more distinctions you make, the more neural pathways that get formed, until at some point both your perception and movement will be noticeably different. To see an obvious example of this, watch an infant as she rolls around on the floor exploring movement. Though her explorations may appear random, what she is doing is making distinctions and thereby adding precision, coordination, and control to her movement. From a neurological perspective, her persistent exploration is akin to tending to an apple tree. Each time she explores, she "sprouts" new branches in the form of neural pathways while simultaneously "pruning" and "weeding out" older, unused ones. The constant sprouting, pruning, and weeding out produces an ever more intricate pattern in her brain. Over time, her perception and movement will become more and more refined. Initially only able to crawl, she will eventually bear the fruits of standing and walking.

What most distinguishes Olympians from most people is how much relative sprouting, pruning, and weeding out they have done. What distinguishes them, in other words, is their ability to make finer distinctions and thereby control with more precision their 630-odd muscles. This edge in control allows them to run with much greater efficiency so that they waste far less energy per stride. Therefore, more energy goes toward propelling them forward, meaning that for every measure of effort they use, they get far greater returns.

Another way to look at distinctions is through the analogy of a race car. An Olympic runner is like a race car whose engine has been finely tuned, wheels aligned to the tiniest fraction of an inch, and indeed, all the proper adjustments painstakingly made such that it runs at the highest level of efficiency. That very same car would run very differently if, however, it had been mistreated, in which case it wouldn't matter what kind of fuel you added, or how hard you stepped on the pedal. Nothing short of a major overhaul would get it running in peak condition.

When you consider that all bodies have the potential to run with higher—and often much higher—efficiency, you begin to realize that how you tune yourself is absolutely vital to how well you run and how good you feel when you're in motion. To return to the race car analogy, you are the mechanic for your own body, and by learning to make new distinctions, you begin the process of fine-tuning yourself. If, on the other hand, you neglect the learning—as you do when you ignore your senses—no amount of effort, green leafy vegetables, or "high-octane" protein powder is going to improve your efficiency.

Perhaps now it is easier to understand what happens when we try to imitate great runners. Lacking their sense-ability, or in other words, their ability to make fine distinctions, we find ourselves unable to perform the way they do. Yet we behave as if increasing our effort will somehow achieve the desired result. Repetition of a flawed performance, however, does not lead to improvement—though it may lead to strain and injury.

Know What You're Doing

If the biggest difference between the greatest and the great, the great and the good, the good and the average is a matter of making finer distinctions through sensing, then it makes sense to sense more of what you are doing. As I mentioned in chapter 7, "To Be or Not To Be," Moshe Feldenkrais is known for saying, "You can't do what you want if you don't know what you are doing." And you don't know what you are doing if you can't sense what you are doing. Knowing, in other words, is sensing.

This means that short of improving your sense-ability, following the conventional route of performing rote exercises, lifting weights, and following simple tips laid out by experts will have a minimal effect on improving the mechanics of your stride. The conventional route will help your stride, in other words, only if what you do can actually be felt while you are running. Surprisingly, following the conventional route may even be detrimental in certain cases, since it tends to further ingrain self-destructive habits. As we saw in chapter 5, "Intention," such habits involve parasitic muscle contractions and stereotyped movement patterns that prevent you from running with more power and ease.

Lifting weights to build stronger muscles, for example, may be beneficial unless the added bulk it imparts to specific muscles goes toward pulling you even more off balance and more off course, thereby adding more stress to your ankles, knees, back, and shoulders. Along with the stress to your joints, the added imbalance could ironically cause you to work even harder in order to keep yourself on course, thereby making running even more laborious. This is why people who lift weights are not necessarily more powerful and fluid in activities that don't involve a dumbbell. Surprisingly, many people in the gym haven't learned to sense and therefore use their bodies in a manner that allows for the force to go where they want it to go. And herein lies the key to improving your stride: in order to use yourself powerfully, you must know what you are doing. And to know what you are doing, you must be able to make distinctions by sensing and feeling what you are doing. The more you can sense what you are doing, the more unified your intention and the greater your power.

So when you really take the time to sense more, you begin to tap into the vast reservoir of power and grace that great runners have been tapping into. By sensing more, your stride actually becomes more like that of an Olympian.

Know Others
(Including Their Anatomical Differences)

Human proportions vary considerably from continent to continent, region to region, and race to race. In parts of Sub-Saharan Africa such as Kenya, for example, people exhibit a higher center of gravity because they have a shorter torso-to-leg ratio. The result is more curvature in their spine. In parts of East Asia such as China and Japan, we see the opposite: people have a lower center of gravity because they possess longer torsos relative to the length of their legs. The result is less curvature in their spine.

People's legs also come in different shapes and sizes, depending on ancestry. The crural index measures the length of the tibia, or shinbone, relative to the femur, or thighbone. Scientists have discovered that people whose ancestors come from the same region tend to exhibit similar crural indexes—which is to say, their legs are proportionally similar.

So what does all this have to do with running?

The anatomical structure of humans by and large determines what kind of posture and patterns of movement best suit them. Someone with a higher center of mass and higher crural index may run more efficiently, for example, using a style that doesn't suit someone with a lower center of mass. It may be more efficient for Kenyans to run by leaning a little forward. But does this mean that it is just as efficient for Norwegians or Japanese to do the same? Someone with entirely different skeletal proportions might not be well suited to leaning forward any more than Catherine Ndereba or any of the other great Kenyan runners might be suited to running very erect. Simply put, your body type will likely require a different style of running in order for you to run as smoothly and powerfully as someone with a different body type. By trying to imitate the Kenyans, you might actually be choosing a less efficient way to run and thereby slowing yourself down. In the process, you would also be missing out on discovering different ways of running that are more ideal for your particular structure.

Anatomical differences aside, there is the important issue of what we think someone is doing compared to what they are actually doing. Obviously, if we want to accurately imitate what someone is doing, we must first accurately know what they are doing. On first glance, Catherine Ndereba and other great Kenyan runners may appear to be leaning forward as they come down the homestretch. Yet are they really leaning forward, or is the pronounced curvature in their spine creating the illusion that they are leaning forward? And if they truly are leaning, from which joints do they lean? If you consider that it's possible to lean from your ankles, hips, any of the twenty-four vertebrae in your spine, or any combination of these, then you can see how the prospect of imitating someone is rife with pitfalls.

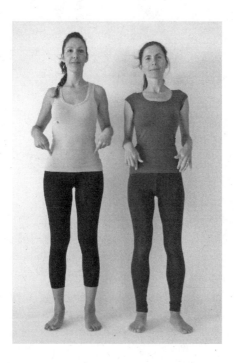

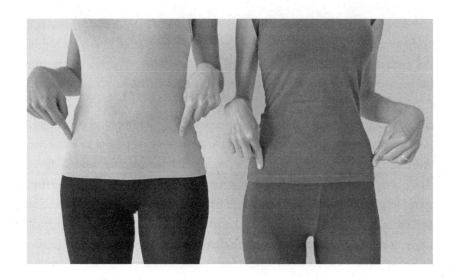

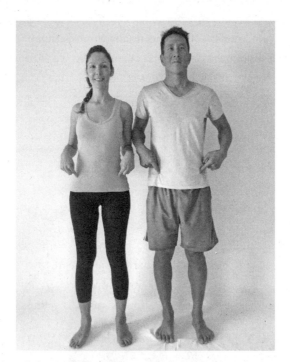

Each person is pointing to the same part of their pelvis. Note that two people can have the same leg length even if one person happens to be taller. Conversely, two people can be the same height even if one has longer legs.

Finally, even if we have figured out precisely what someone else is doing, being able to do it ourselves is often much harder than it looks. For example, the vast majority of people who are instructed to lean will very rarely do it in the same manner as someone like Catherine Ndereba (assuming she leans while running). Instead, they will lean by utilizing all of their particular sensorimotor habits rather than the habits of a great Kenyan runner. It's not for a lack of effort that they are unable to accurately carry out the task, but that everybody's sensorimotor habits arise from their own individual sense-abilities. Thus, if you don't have the sense-abilities of a great Kenyan runner, you won't be able to move like a great Kenyan runner, no matter how hard you try. When attempting to lean forward like the Kenyans, some people will consequently collapse their chest forward, forcing them to crane their neck back, while others will hunch their back, causing other distortions in the spine. Such inaccurate imitations will naturally produce completely different results, none of which is likely to achieve the desired gain in power.

Obviously, the problem here is not that we don't know how to lean forward, but that we don't really know how to do it in the manner of Catherine Ndereba. In other words, if I lean forward but lack the requisite sense-ability of a Kenyan track star, I will do it in my particular way—that is, using my particular movement habits—which is quite different from the way the Kenyan track star does it. And believe it or not, something so simple as leaning forward has as many variations as there are people on the planet.[1]

Posture: "Oops, I Swallowed a Yardstick!"

Whether or not any of us tries to lean the way a Kenyan track star appears to be leaning, many people agree that it's important run with a "straight" back. Many people also believe that straightness, or what is deemed "good posture"—whether for sitting, standing, or running—must be imposed on

---

[1] In their best-selling book, *ChiRunning: A Revolutionary Approach to Effortless, Injury-Free Running* (New York: Fireside, 2004), Danny and Katherine Dreyer have developed some creative exercises that may help you to lean forward without collapsing your spine.

an otherwise crooked body. This being the case, where does the crookedness come from?

Our collective obsession with posture is itself revealing to how the dominant culture views life. Posture comes from the Latin word *positura*, meaning "station" or "position," which presupposes a static and therefore unchanging state. Yet in order to maintain our station or position, we must ignore our senses, since paying attention to them, as we shall see, would mean constantly changing our station or position. And unfortunately, if we ignore our senses, we must rely on outside sources to define what is good and what is bad.

Obviously, life is not static, as the word *posture* would lead us to believe. Rather, it is perpetually in flux and thus perpetually asking us to adapt our movement to suit the task at hand, be it running, getting out of a chair, or simply standing in line at the checkout counter. And whereas stasis insinuates predictability and some level of confinement, adaptability is itself freedom.

For those of us with postural issues, we are in effect experiencing confinement created by our habits. To break out of the prison, it won't help to force "good" posture on ourselves. In fact, we actually experience the opposite of freedom when we attempt to "sit up straight," "stand tall," or otherwise walk around with a "straight" back. We intuitively know something isn't right because trying to be "straight" usually doesn't feel so good. In fact, after a very short time—and we can normally only hold it for a matter of seconds—it feels tiresome and uncomfortable. Sit up straighter right now and see how long you end up staying there. If you're like me and most people I know, it will be ten seconds or less before a distraction will lead you back to your habitual posture.

The reason that forcing changes in posture doesn't feel good is because you are attempting to impose something new on top of something else that doesn't just magically disappear. You end up with two minds jockeying for position in one body, or to use an earlier analogy, you end up with offense and defense playing against each other. Because the old habitual patterns are still there, in other words, forcing something on top of it is a form of suppression. You can literally feel the internal struggle through increased effort.

We can usually sense when people around us are trying to imitate good posture simply because they look stiff and uncomfortable. In trying to be straight, they look like they are trying to fit themselves into a mold—perhaps a bit like soldiers who are standing at attention. Moshe Feldenkrais himself commented on how we are all familiar with people among us who have swallowed a yardstick. We are familiar because we ourselves do it from time to time when we are trying to impress others.

Freedom

Ideally, the human body is not static like the frozen spine of a drill sergeant standing at attention, but active, like that of a Olympic runner who can at one moment bound powerfully down the track, and the next moment gracefully bend down to tie her shoe. Because the bounding and bending require very different uses of her spine and indeed her entire body from head to toe, the stasis implicit in the word *posture* is misleading.

Realizing this, Moshe Feldenkrais coined a more adaptive term for how we could be carrying ourselves as we go through life. *Acture,* which comes from the Latin root *actus,* meaning "a doing," insinuates action and change. Since Feldenkrais believed that the way we carry ourselves could become more and more of an active process, keeping ourselves static actually prevents us from moving well.[2]

For Moshe Feldenkrais, the concept of acture is meant not only to insinuate action but moreover actions we most often carry out. This means that how I normally carry myself is simply an outward manifestation of the movement patterns I use most often. So if I spend eight hours a day hunched over a desk and craning my chin forward in order to see my computer screen, the hunching and craning movement patterns may eventually become dominant—even when I am not at my desk. Conversely, the more

---

[2] It is important to note that everybody does, in fact, adapt to some degree to the task at hand. The issue Feldenkrais makes, however, is that few of us adapt to a high degree. Thus, we may continue to keep our backs straight even when it's not appropriate, such as when bending down to tie our shoelaces.

my daily repertoire reflects a sense-able adaptation to everyday tasks, the more efficient, graceful, and powerful my acture becomes.

All of this is to say that good acture (or, if you prefer, "good posture") is the result of increasing my movement options, paying more attention to how I am doing what I am doing, and otherwise acquiring greater sense-ability in everyday life. Good acture, in other words, comes naturally through tuning in to my senses, rather than tuning out of them through force and willpower. If my daily activities include training in a way that allows me to discover more powerful, coordinated, and graceful ways to carry my body down the track, then the accrued movement patterns will make me taller, more powerful, and coordinated even when I'm not training. You'll notice, for example, how effortlessly tall and erect Olympic track athletes stand and walk. They aren't trying to be tall; they simply are tall as a result of their movement habits. Conversely, the more I employ movement patterns that are not linked with greater sense-ability, and consequently not linked to more power, coordination, and fluidity, the heavier, less coordinated, and possibly shorter I will feel.[3] I cannot simply imbibe power, coordination, and fluidity and thus magically absorb good acture. Good acture can only come through one avenue: sensing more.

Here again, we return to the fact that in order to successfully imitate (in this case "good" acture), I need to sense and feel and therefore know what's happening inside myself. I cannot artificially impose good acture on myself and expect to look, feel, and move like the people I am trying to imitate. To do so is to look for a shortcut that doesn't exist. The potent acture that Olympians carry is a natural result of finely tuning the race car, so to

---

[3] I believe that getting shorter as we age is not simply a function of bone loss, but concomitant with the ways that we habitually carry ourselves. The people who grow shorter at a faster rate are likely those who carry faulty acture. It's encouraging to note here that it is actually possible to stand taller with age if you continue to improve your sense-ability and thereby improve your acture. During my Feldenkrais training, I was astonished to discover myself going through a "growth spurt" where I literally grew taller. Even though the objective gain in height was minimal—probably a fraction of an inch over four years—the subjective feeling made me feel ten feet tall. The feeling of standing tall, for the first time in my life, in other words, made me feel like a whole new person—more empowered than I had felt in decades.

speak. Attempting to copy their potent acture by leaning forward or forcing myself to stand tall, on the other hand, is like stepping on the gas, hoping that sheer willpower and force will produce a superior performance. Good acture, in other words, does not cause my movement repertoire to suddenly expand. Rather, it is a result of the movement repertoire that already exists. Simply standing "straighter" or leaning forward, then, does not automatically cause me to have the movement repertoire and therefore the powerful stride of the great Kenyan runners. Increasing my sense-ability and thereby adding movement patterns to my repertoire, however, does allow me to run with more power and does affect my acture in a positive way.

Are You Saying Imitation Is Bad?

Imitation itself is not the trap per se. Rather, it is the assumption that (1) we know ourselves; (2) we know others.

Does this mean we should never imitate somebody else?

No. What it means is that if it's to be of benefit to us, we need to pay attention to how imitating someone's movement feels in our own bodies. If we want to be more accurate in imitating movement patterns, we need to start discovering, first of all, what it is we are actually doing in our own bodies. Then and only then will we be able to accurately discover what it is that other people are doing in theirs.

The pitfall here is that we normally possess an idea of what we are doing that bears little resemblance to what it is we are actually doing. The same goes for watching other people. We think we know what they are doing when in fact all we possess is a crude approximation—often wrought with illusion—of their way of moving. Whether or not we are accurate in our ideas of ourselves or in approximating others is left to us to discern through meticulous exploration and frequently asking the Three Cardinal Questions.

As a final note to this chapter, you'll notice that not all world-class runners lean forward when they run. And not all of them run as tall and erect as someone like the great 400-meter champion Michael Johnson. In fact, most do neither, for one very good reason: it doesn't feel good to them. This is not to say trying to imitate Catherine Ndereba's forward alignment or Michael

Johnson's straight up-and-down carriage is wrong, but rather that imitating any particular style is not a necessary key to running more efficiently.

To get a good idea of how the position of your spine—leaning or not—affects how much power you have going up stairs and up hills, go to Lesson 10, "Standing Tall Without Trying to Stand Tall."

9

Who Turned Up
the Gravity?

*Gravity is, if you will, the universe's nearest approximation to
what theologians might call an immanent deity: namely, a God
that is universal, ubiquitous, law-giving, and all powerful.*

—THOMAS HANNA, *THE BODY OF LIFE:*
CREATING NEW PATHWAYS FOR SENSORY
AWARENESS AND FLUID MOVEMENT

Life is anything but static. Yet modern culture leads us to believe that it is,
causing us to do all we can to resist change and cling to our habits. Unfortunately, our habits don't always serve us well.

Perhaps the only thing that remains static is gravity. The earth exerts
a constant pull, yet we perceive the constancy as change. We describe this
change with words like "light" or "heavy," "powerful" or "weak," "fluid" or
"jerky," "grounded" or "ungrounded." Though we may often feel like someone is turning the gravity dial up or down, it is not gravity that is changing,
but rather our relationship with it.

Why would our relationship with gravity continue to change?

Because to be alive is to move, and to move requires that you find a way to maintain your balance. Simply lifting your leg requires a whole series of adjustments in order to stabilize certain joints and keep you from falling on your face. In order for some part of you to move, other parts have to provide a stable foundation for that movement. Moving one part of your body, in other words, is not really moving just that one part. It is moving that part in concert with the entire rest of your body—or simply put, it is your whole body moving at once, though it may appear as if only one part is in motion. One way to look at it is like this: if I reach forward with my foot, is it my foot that is reaching forward, or the rest of my body that is reaching backward with respect to my foot? For that matter, where does my foot begin and where does it end?

This is why, when we are running, one leg always goes backward as the other goes forward. This is also why the faster you run, the more you pump your arms. As we saw earlier, it isn't just the legs that are moving. Everything above your waist can be used to support or even initiate what is happening below your waist. Imagine running with your arms bound to your sides by rope and you will immediately have a sense of how important the arms are for maintaining balance and increasing power.

Gravity, Effort, and the
Three Cardinal Questions

Answering the Three Cardinal Questions is a way to measure our relationship with gravity. The amount of effort we need to exert in order to do anything describes the degree to which gravity has become our friend or our enemy. Generally speaking, the less refined our sense-ability, the less efficiently we move.[1] And the less efficiently we move, the heavier we feel, and therefore the more effort we need to exert in order to do whatever it is we want to do.

---

[1] Of course, to be efficient, your sense-abilities must relate on some level to the activity at hand. While a concert pianist will have highly developed sense-abilities for playing the piano, such sense-abilities will probably not translate easily to running or swimming powerfully. Likewise, while Olympic runners possess sense-abilities that relate to efficient propulsion on land, they probably won't help much for swimming or playing the piano.

Efficiency is, in fact, reflected in every aspect of living, from how you walk down the street to how you stand while waiting in line at the supermarket checkout counter to how you position your head when you gaze (read, stare fixedly) at your cell phone. It is even reflected in the way you breathe. For example, do you ever feel like you can't get enough air, as if someone is pressing on your chest? Any difficulty in breathing means that you are not only working harder in order to do what should come naturally, but getting less oxygen in the process. In many cases, unintentional constriction in your chest, lower back, and abdomen literally holds your breath in. The question you might then ask is, "Who is holding my breath?"

Everything in life can, in fact, be linked to effort. When we say things like "I'm walking on clouds," "She's got the weight of the world on her shoulders," or "He sucked the air out of the room," we are, whether consciously or unconsciously, giving indication to the amount of effort we need to exert in order to accomplish a particular task. If, for example, I'm walking on clouds, I will feel lighter, and thus less effort is going into each step. Likewise, if I feel like I have extra weight on my shoulders, I will feel like it requires more effort just to stand erect. And if someone has "sucked the air out of the room," it indicates that breathing has become more laborious and thus more effortful.

It is important to note that statements like these also suggest the intrinsic link between feelings, emotions, and acture. Thus, if you're walking on clouds, you're probably not feeling depressed or experiencing a bout of road rage. And if you're hanging your head and dragging your feet, it's certainly not due to a sense of pride, contentment, or fulfillment. The mind-body unity, which can also be thought of as the feeling-emotion-acture unity, dictates, in fact, that each and every feeling and emotion you experience will correspond to a particular acture or family of actures, each of which will in turn influence your quality of movement. Thus, at any given moment you will feel lighter or heavier, stronger or weaker, more balanced or less balanced in the physical sense, depending on what feelings and emotions are coursing through you in the psychological sense.

This relationship between feeling, emotion, and acture is one reason coaches, sportscasters, and athletes place so much emphasis on momentum and morale changes during the heat of the battle. When the momentum shifts in, say, a football game, it means that one team has suddenly lost its emotional edge, as will be manifest in the players' expressions and acture. Likewise, players who have lost their morale will display the inner turmoil not only on their faces but through their entire body. Consequently, they will likely not only feel but actually become weaker and more fatigued, or perhaps even less agile and less able to respond appropriately. It follows that unless these players can change their emotional state, they will be stuck in acture and therefore movement patterns that are less efficient, less powerful, and more effortful.[2]

In short, each and every feeling you feel and emotion you experience will play a unique role in affecting your acture in some subtle to obvious way. Feelings and emotions you possess (or that possess you) at any given moment will consequently have some subtle to profound influence on the quality of your every movement and thereby influence everything from your sense of balance to the quality of your stride. With this in consideration, it's no wonder why, in the last few decades, sports psychology has emerged as a legitimate subcategory of psychology and why, since time immemorial,

---

[2] Players who have lost their morale will appear to have given up, and during a game this is considered to be bad. I consider giving up to be neither intrinsically bad nor good, but simply a necessary part of learning. Great innovations and improvements often come after we've engaged in an intensive period of work and "given up" to rest for a while. We often hear stories of people coming up with new ideas while relaxing in the bathtub or somewhere else. Richard Feynman, for example, first got the idea for what was to become his Nobel Prize–winning thesis while sitting in the university dining hall: "He was eating in the student cafeteria when someone tossed a dinner plate into the air—a Cornell cafeteria plate with the university seal imprinted on one rim—and in the instant of its flight he experienced what he long afterward considered an epiphany. As the plate spun, it wobbled. Because of the insignia he could see that the spin and the wobble were not quite in synchrony. Yet just in that instant it seemed to him—or was it his physicist's intuition?—that the two rotations were related. He had told himself he was going to play, so he tried to work out the problem on paper." James Gleick, *The Life and Science of Richard Feynman* (New York: Pantheon, 1992), 227–28.

athletes themselves often perform rituals to get "psyched up" (some of which may play an added role of "psyching out" their opponents), before competition.

You Cannot Laugh and Clench Your Jaw at the Same Time

If feelings and emotions have a direct bearing on acture, it follows that any given feeling or emotion can either detract from or aid in exploring a particular movement or performing a particular action. The type of acture associated with clenching your jaw, for example, which could arise from any number of feelings or emotions, including anger, frustration, impatience, irritation, or anxiety, may aid in preventing you from getting knocked out when getting hit on the chin by someone else's fist (as in the sport of boxing), but it probably won't contribute to improving your 10,000-meter time. This is because the type of acture appropriate for protecting yourself from a concussive blow to the head is not necessarily appropriate for generating an easy and powerful stride.

Because feelings and emotions influence acture, they also influence movement. For if acture could be considered one frame within that motion picture of continuous movement we call "life," movement could be considered the collection of those frames into a contiguous whole. Obviously, you can't change one single frame without changing an entire scene. This is why, upon observing students grinding their teeth, holding their breath, or otherwise clutching onto dear life during a lesson, I often look for ways to make them laugh. As laughter erupts, jaws release their viselike grip, chests and bellies fill with air, and other parasitic patterns begin to disappear: a tightly held shoulder, for example, begins to let go, a clenched fist opens into an offering palm, a hard stare softens into a calm gaze.

Note that this is not an admonition of anyone for ever having had anything other than relaxed, free, and happy thoughts. If we were to try to extinguish "negative" thoughts, feelings, and emotions, and thereby arrive at happiness or relaxation through something like positive thinking, we run the danger of becoming the person who swallows the proverbial yardstick in order to stand straighter.[3] We run the danger, in other words, of simply imposing a knee-jerk correction on ourselves and likely suppressing our real thoughts, feelings, and emotions as a result.[4]

---

[3] I hesitate to label any emotion "negative" (hence the quotation marks), precisely because popular culture has deemed negativity as something to be excised, diminished, and ultimately disappeared from view, if not existence. I believe that all emotions, whether deemed "positive" or "negative," are intrinsic to being fully alive. When a culture or subculture develops an allergy to particular feelings and emotions, those feelings and emotions will likely become suppressed among the populace. And just as trying to force "good posture" on ourselves doesn't make the old habits go away, trying to force "positive emotions" on ourselves will not make the feelings and emotions lying beneath a veneer of positivity magically disappear. Furthermore, suppression does not come without a cost: "Rigidity in man cannot be obtained without suppressing some activity for which he has the capacity. Thus, continuous and unreserved adherence to any principle, good or bad, means suppressing some function continuously. This suppression cannot be practiced with impunity for any length of time." Moshe Feldenkrais, *Body and Mature Behavior: A Study of Anxiety, Sex, Gravitation & Learning* (Madison, CT: International Universities Press, 1992), 13. When channeled toward constructive purposes, "negative" emotions such as anger and indignation can actually have a very positive effect. One could go as far as to say that many, most, and perhaps all of the progressive political economic changes that have occurred in the last two centuries have sprouted from mass anger and indignation in the face of injustice.

[4] While there may be a kernel of truth lying somewhere beneath the murky waters of positive thinking and the myriad forms of psychological and spiritual counseling that have been popularized by the self-help industry, such well-intended messages can have a toxic and even self-defeating effect if doled out without consideration and empathy for each individual's unique circumstances—ones that may, in fact, be nigh impossible to change or break out of, no matter how positive or spiritual the individual. Moreover, while positive thinking and other recipes for self-improvement normally focus strictly on the individual, they conveniently sidestep the deep structural problems facing society—structures, incidentally, that play a crucial role in exacerbating or even creating some of the individual problems they claim to address. Philosopher Charles Eisenstein demystifies some of the thinking behind New Age mysticism in two succinct sentences: "When I was broke a couple of years ago, I remember feeling annoyed when well-meaning spiritual friends told me my problem was 'an attitude of scarcity.' When the economy of an entire country like Latvia or Greece collapses and millions go bankrupt, shall we blame it on their attitudes? What about poor, hungry children—do they have scarcity mentality too?" Charles Eisenstein, *Sacred Economics: Money, Gift and Society in the Age of Transition* (Berkeley, CA: North Atlantic Books, 2011), 121. Religious studies scholar Huston Smith addresses the issue even more plainly: "To shout from the safe shore to a drowning person, 'Chin up!' is an insult." Philip Cousineau, ed., *The Way Things Are: Conversations with Huston Smith on the Spiritual Life* (Berkeley, CA: University of California Press, 2003), 72.

Turning Down Gravity

The relationship between acture, movement patterns, and effort is why it can be so enlivening to improve your sense-abilities. Improved sense-abilities generally help to improve your relationship with gravity, thereby improving your breathing patterns and making you feel lighter—as if Mother Nature just turned down the gravity dial.

The relationship described above is also one reason why Olympic coaches stress the importance of maintaining your form when you start to fatigue. Each minute change in form can do either one of two things: (1) pull you off balance, causing you to immediately become less efficient because you consequently need to devote more of your energy to simply staying in balance; or (2) make you more balanced, meaning more of your energy goes toward propelling you forward, rather than in some undesired direction.

The difficulty here is that when you get tired, it becomes more difficult to control your muscles and therefore more likely that you will begin to lose your form and thereby unwittingly increase your workload. To some degree, losing form is a natural part of muscle fatigue because when you start to tire, it is more difficult to control your movement. But this doesn't mean that your movement has to be totally out of control.

When some people begin to tire, their form really falls apart. I am quite familiar with this phenomenon because I used to clench my shoulders and swing my head wildly whenever I started getting tired. This created enormous stress on my body because it caused more energy to be diverted toward propelling me in the wrong direction, which forced me to spend even more energy to keep myself running in the right direction. Without realizing it, I had done the equivalent of plopping a sandbag on my shoulders—and I did it at a time when I was least able to deal with added stress.

So when your form falls apart, you are actually giving yourself more work. And this means that the more your form disintegrates, the more effort you need to exert to stay on track—and literally stay on the track, because parasitic muscle tension may be pulling you off the track.

Looking at it this way, effort is a measure of the quality of your stride. The more efficient you are, the more propulsion you get per measure of effort. Or, put more simply, higher efficiency means that you can travel the same distance and do so faster, while exerting less effort. Conversely, the less efficient your stride, the more proverbial sandbags you are carrying on your shoulders, and therefore the more effort you need to expend.

This is not to say that great runners don't use effort. They exert a tremendous amount. But for each amount, they literally cover more ground because less of their work goes toward piling sandbags on their shoulders and more of it goes toward propelling their bodies forward. As a result, each individual stride will propel them much farther than that of the average jogger. And this is why they look so light when they are running—as if they are floating on air.

To maintain better form, even as you fatigue, it helps to practice tuning into specific points in your body from time to time. Then, when you get tired or are pushing it down the homestretch, it will be much easier to focus on these points. For example, you could focus on keeping the back of your neck long, reaching for the sky with the center top of your head, or rolling off particular metatarsals. Lesson 14, "Water Jugs, Furniture, and Other Things to Carry on Your Head," addresses the former two, and many of the lessons from the "Throwing the Ball" series address rolling off different parts of your foot. Whatever places you choose, every now and then, practice bringing your attention to them while running.

10

Following Instructions: Where Do My Knees Begin?

As social scientists Joseph Henrich, Steve Heine, and Ara Noren-
zayan express it, most of our understanding of human psychology
is based on subjects who may be described by the acronym WEIRD:
from Western, educated, industrialized, rich, and democratic societies.

—JARED DIAMOND, *THE WORLD UNTIL*
YESTERDAY: WHAT CAN WE LEARN
FROM TRADITIONAL SOCIETIES?

Over the years I have noticed two vital questions that few of us ask ourselves when being given "expert" advice:

Should I follow the advice?

How should I follow the advice?

Before following someone else's advice, it is a good idea to examine the
foundation upon which the advice is based. This is because behind every
instruction lies a series of assumptions of which even the advice-givers may

be unaware. Look closely at any piece of writing from a physics textbook to the *New York Times* to this running book and you will find a world of assumptions. This isn't a bad thing. We need them in order to make sense of, and thereby organize, our world. You could say that assumptions are a way of simplifying the world into something more manageable. They allow us to make generalizations such as "Touching a hot stove hurts," or "Getting enough sleep puts me in a better mood." And in this manner, assumptions form the basis of what we have already learned.

What we have learned in the past, however, is not always appropriate for the present. And this means that learning—which only takes place in the present—could be considered the active process of uncovering assumptions—specifically false ones.

Because assumptions are generally made on an unconscious level, it is difficult to notice them. The average person in the modern industrialized world, for example, assumes that the terrain on which she walks is completely flat and even. This is evident in her gait and explains why she is more likely to stumble when she meets an unexpected crack in the sidewalk as compared to someone who is used to navigating uneven terrain. The assumption itself is neither good nor bad but a natural part of the way the human nervous system adapts to its environment. And in this way, assumptions may serve us, but only to the degree that the terrain never changes.

As humans, we all trip over literal and proverbial cracks in the sidewalk from time to time. Doing so affords us the opportunity to really start paying attention to the terrain. But as I mentioned earlier, paying attention requires slowing down—a difficult endeavor when you live in a world where everything is speeding up. Thus, we are caught in what appears to be a dilemma. To keep up with the world, I have to speed up. But to learn from my mistakes, I need to slow down. Which do I choose?

To slow down is in a sense to speed up because by taking my time, I gain all the clarity, accuracy, and precision that come with learning. From a neurophysiological standpoint, slowing down gives my nervous system the opportunity to absorb much more information, make distinctions, and fine-tune my motor control so that when I choose to speed up again, my movement will be more precise and less hampered by parasitic muscle contractions. To revisit an earlier analogy, if I want to drive to Chicago and I live in San Francisco, heading west will not get me to my destination any faster, no matter how hard I step on the gas.

Another way to look at it is that by refusing to slow down, I am liable to make the same mistakes over and over. For refusing to slow down is in many cases equivalent to refusing to pay attention. And to those of us who refuse to pay attention, our constant stumbling will remain a mystery. We will continue driving into the ocean and blame the car, not realizing that it's our lack of attentiveness that has brought us to where we are.

How Should I Follow Instructions?

This is another way of saying, "What do the instructions really mean?" For example, what does it mean when someone says, "lift your knees higher"?[1]

These questions may appear to be silly because we think we understand simple instructions. The problem is, very few instructions are as simple as they first appear. As I mentioned earlier, "lean forward when you run" is a very complex instruction requiring you to really understand body mechanics and differences between your body and the body of the person you're trying to imitate. In the end, this seemingly simple instruction turns out to be quite ambiguous. The common dictum among track coaches, "Lift your knees higher," is similarly rife with pitfalls.

From a conventional coaching perspective, lifting your knees higher means just that. So whenever coaches told me to lift my knees, it's what I tried to do. What we didn't realize, however, is that as with leaning forward, there is an untold number of ways to lift your knees higher. Furthermore, none of us knew that the simple instruction to lift your knees higher contains three major

---

[1] I heard this phrase over and over when I was a serious runner. The assumption here is that by lifting your knees higher you will run faster. Yet, if you watch films of Alberto Salazar, who won three consecutive New York City Marathons back in the early 1980s, or Michael Johnson, who dominated the 200- and 400-meter dash over the course of two Olympiads, you may begin to question such advice. Obviously, the assumption that lifting your knees higher makes you faster remains true only some of the time.

assumptions: (1) that there is only one right way to lift your knees higher; (2) that I would be able to figure out how to do it that one right way; and (3) that by doing it that one right way I would actually become a better runner.

Try it now if you like: run down the hallway and lift your knees higher than you normally do. Is it relatively more or less effort? If it is more, how long do you think you could sustain that increased level of effort? Do you feel lighter or heavier? How do your back and neck feel? Take some time to really notice.

Operator

Giving and following instructions is like giving and receiving messages in the children's game called "Operator." With several children sitting in a circle, the game begins when one child whispers a short message to the one next to her. The second child in turn passes the message on to the child next to him. The message goes around in the circle until it returns to the first child. Simple enough.

Yet the results reveal that passing a message is not so simple. In fact, the whole fun in the game is discovering how the message returns to the original sender and bears little or no resemblance to the original. The amusement, in other words, is in how the content gets to be totally and unintentionally revised. While each child has tried her best to pass on the original message, each has unwittingly changed it through her own interpretive skills.

Interpretation is not only limited to children playing a game, but it is part and parcel of all communication, including that between adults. This means that each of us, regardless of age, will interpret the same instructions in a different fashion. Each of us, in other words, will choose one among a countless number of ways to perform the instruction. Thus, even the simplest instructions will yield different results for different people.

So the question then becomes, how do you get an accurate interpretation?

The answer is, you generally don't, because you are interpreting the instructions through your ability to understand them. And this ability rests on the depth of your sense-ability. If you happen to already possess the requisite sense-ability that would allow you to move as the instructor intends, then you will get a fairly accurate interpretation. The problem is few of us possess the requisite sense-ability at the outset, and if we did, we probably wouldn't be looking for help to begin with.

This fact notwithstanding, you can still reap benefits from following (interpreting) instructions, if you view all learning as a process and take each new instruction as an experiment. In this case, what you are looking for is how each interpretation of each new instruction affects the way you feel. Pay attention to the process, in other words, and you will maximize your learning and improvement.[2] And this brings us back to the Three Cardinal Questions. Here they are again:

How much effort does it take to move from one position to the next (and therefore, how can you minimize the effort)?

How solid is your connection with the ground?

Does it feel good?

As I elucidated earlier, asking the Three Cardinal Questions assures that you are staying in tune with your senses and therefore your mind, which makes you much more likely to become engrossed in the process rather than fixating on the end result. In this manner, asking the Three Cardinal Questions when interpreting any instructions not only prevents you from doing damage to yourself, but dramatically enhances your learning and your ability to feel pleasure.

In contrast, by fixating on "getting it done" or "getting results," and thereby not staying in process, you are not only more likely to get injured but less likely to improve. What's more, performing in a rote way—which is what happens when you are not being mindful—you will have taken the fun out of learning. Indeed, you will have taken the learning out of learning, thereby turning your directed actions into a boring and possibly self-destructive chore.

---

[2] Note that the instructions contained in this book are designed to cut out as many variables as possible so as to make the interpretation easier. Learning occurs most rapidly when your mind only has to deal with one or two variables at once. Too many and the mind gets overwhelmed. Scientists commonly use the principle of minimizing variables, knowing that having too many prevents them from drawing reliable conclusions. Athletes and martial artists do this in form of simple drills that get more complex as they master more skills. Watch a varsity basketball or soccer practice sometime and you will get an idea of what it means to minimize variables.

The Complexity of the Human Body

Another reason following even simple instructions is wrought with so many pitfalls has to do with the underlying assumption that people will follow them in a way that deepens their sense-abilities, thereby creating more efficient movement patterns. Those who are giving the instructions, in other words, unwittingly assume that by following their advice, people will discover new and more efficient ways of moving that reside outside of their habitual patterns. Recall that if you continue to use your old movement patterns, you won't improve in any fundamental way, and what's more, you will end up practicing all of your habits. By practicing your habits, you won't, in other words, learn. This works fine if, like Catherine Ndereba, you already possess good running habits, but not so well if you don't (though even world-class runners can benefit from discovering new movement patterns). To go back to an earlier analogy, practicing habits is for most of us akin to fortifying our defense, or in other words, perfecting the art of self-sabotage.

Why it is so difficult to accurately follow instructions has to do with the complexity of the human body and mind. Though many instructions appear to be simple, each and every one invariably presents the nervous system with an overwhelming number of choices. How do you move some 630 muscles attached to over 200 bones and controlling roughly 230 joints vis-à-vis an ever-changing environment, in a way that corresponds to what your coach or author intended?

If you consider that, in combination, all of these bones, joints, and muscles present a potential for movement that is virtually limitless, you can begin to understand why the human mind dwarfs even the most sophisticated supercomputer in its ability to integrate patterns. And you can also understand how easy it is to miss the mark.

The Knee Bone's Connected to the Thigh Bone; the Thigh Bone's Connected to the ...

Because your knee is connected to your shin, it is inextricably linked to the movement of your shin and everything below your shin—namely your foot and ankle. In addition, your knee is connected above to your thighbone, which is inextricably linked to the movement of the pelvis. Your pelvis itself acts like the Grand Central Station of bodily movement because it is the central nexus that links all the pieces together. Not only does your pelvis help to integrate the right and left sides of your body, but it connects the upper and lower half and front and back as well. If you were to break down the force vectors that travel through your pelvis with each movement you make, it would look like a massive circuit board with seemingly endless bundles of circuits going to every part of the body.

Looking at the body in this relativistic way, you can begin to see that when something goes up, something else has to go down. And when something goes forward, something else must go backward. Indeed, when something goes in one direction, something else must go in another. Newtonian physics makes another appearance here. Look at the form of good runners and you will notice that when the right knee lifts, it doesn't do so in isolation. The entire body is moving relative to the knee: the left shoulder and arm simultaneously reach forward, the left hip extends backward, and the right shoulder and arm pump backward. And here we run into a conundrum: is it the right knee going forward that causes the rest of the body to react and move in their particular ways, or is it the entire rest of the body that is driving the right knee forward? What is the cause and what is the effect?

By focusing our attention on the knees, my coaches and I unwittingly treated them as the cause. And by doing so, we neglected how the rest of my body played a role in my stride. Would it have been better to look at some other part of the body as the cause?

Symbiosis Versus Cause and Effect

Rather than looking at movement in the conventional way—as independently moving parts—I believe it is much more instructive to see your body as a unified whole in which each part is inextricably linked with the entire rest of you—not only neurologically through sensing and feeling (as we saw in chapter 8, "Imitation"), but biomechanically through force vectors, gravity, and the flow of life or qi.

Cause and effect, which is the conventional way of looking at how the universe works, harks back to the reductionistic way of breaking the world down into discrete, independently moving parts. But what of the possibility that our "discrete parts" actually work symbiotically such that one movement is not strictly the cause of another? If this were the case, then we could begin to see how each muscle and bone plays a reciprocal role in how the entire rest of our body moves. From this perspective, the way I use my left shoulder could play a major role in how I move my right knee, and vice versa. Even the way I use my left big toe could have a significant impact on how I carry my head, and vice versa. Parts that are seemingly removed and distant from each other, in other words, are not so removed or distant when we begin to understand biomechanics as a symbiotic phenomenon.

Symbiosis is not a new concept. The Bagua precepts state that if the center moves, the extremities move, and if the extremities move, the center moves. Bagua could, in this manner, be seen as a search for unification, the practice of which is to unify movement within one's body, and thereby unify intention within one's mind.

Powerful running follows the same precepts even if running coaches and running books don't explicitly state this. Generally speaking, the more powerful and graceful a movement feels, the more you are using yourself as a unified whole in which the "parts" work cooperatively. The less powerful and graceful you feel, the more likely you are moving like a machine whose parts are not cooperating.

All of the lessons in appendix B address symbiosis. Try any one of them now to have an embodied sense of how your body can work as a unified whole.

11

There Are No Shortcuts, No Secrets, No Magic Pills

[Cassius Clay] was just ordinary, and I doubt whether any scout would have thought much of him in his first year. About a year later, though, you could see that the little smart aleck—I mean, he's always been sassy—had a lot of potential.... He was a kid willing to make the sacrifices necessary to achieve something worthwhile in sports. I realized it was almost impossible to discourage him. He was easily the hardest worker of any kid I ever taught.

—JOE MARTIN, MUHAMMAD ALI'S
FIRST BOXING COACH

When you get a black belt ranking it doesn't mean you've gotten a foot in the door. It means you have learned how to find the doorknob.

—DAVE LOWRY, *TRADITIONS: ESSAYS
ON THE JAPANESE MARTIAL ARTS
AND WAYS*

In Hollywood films, the novice pipsqueak trains furiously for a few weeks of cinematic glory compressed into ninety seconds of high-octane, sweat-filled sequences. Then, against all odds, and backed by the London Symphony Orchestra, he or she defeats the seasoned champion.

That's why it's called fiction.

In our hurry-up world we expect too much too soon. Ours is a culture of delusion and dilettantism.

As the chapter title states, there are no shortcuts. Talent may exist, yet those with it do not fundamentally improve unless they put in their time. This is true of everybody from Michelangelo to Muhammad Ali.

If the previous statement appears to contradict the idea of working less in order to increase sense-ability, rest assured, it doesn't. Working less against yourself does not mean hardly working at all. It simply means working more intelligently so that more of your effort goes to where you want it to go.

Jane's Story[1]

Jane normally showed up for my weekly Taichi class after having spent the morning riding her bicycle. "I'm looking for something meditative and noncompetitive," she said on her first day, before announcing that she had just ridden 26.8 miles (apparently she had an odometer on her bicycle). Like most avid cyclists I know, Jane had muscular thighs and well-defined calf muscles. And like most athletes I know, she assumed that one kind of strength could be easily morphed into another—that, for instance, the kind needed to pedal a bicycle across country roads would translate easily into the kind needed to practice Taichi.

Of course, most people assume that you don't even need strength to practice Taichi. Few people, in fact, take the art very seriously because it has become stereotyped as a slow motion sequence performed by old

---

[1] Like John, the character in chapter 2, "The Hurried Runner," Jane is also fictional, even if her traits are drawn from people that I know (including the one who looks back at me from the mirror every morning).

people. In my classes, however, students of all ages quickly discover that movements done slowly and with great precision can be very challenging. Even attending athletes have been surprised to discover that Taichi involves strengthening their bodies in ways with which they were initially unfamiliar. Regardless of their physical aptitude, I let students know that strengthening their body in new and varied ways takes learning and therefore time, exploration, and effort. Strength, I tell them, can be thought of as a skill that can be learned, just like any other skill.

Unmoved by this idea, Jane would express renewed shock at the beginning of each class that a "simple" Taichi warm-up could be so challenging to someone with her tree-trunk legs. Predictably, renewed shock meant renewed excuses. During her first class, for example, Jane let the class know that she could leg press more than most of her peers. "My legs are really very strong," she reassured us several times while struggling with the basic stances. I nodded in acknowledgment, noting that doing the leg press and practicing Taichi require categorically different uses of the body.

As a teacher, I'm mostly interested in how my students are able to learn and mostly uninterested in how proficient they claim to be. I don't need them to boast about their skills when their acture is already speaking volumes as soon as they walk through the door. Furthermore, a few minutes of going through the warm-ups is often more than enough to reveal their level of competence. Moreover, you cannot be performing and exploring both at the same time. So if a student is busy showing off or otherwise in performance mode, she is missing out on valuable learning.

On her eighth, and what was to be final, day of class, Jane arrived as confident as ever. "I rode 30.4 miles this morning," she announced cheerfully. Sadly, trying to convince the class of her physical prowess continued to prevent her from paying attention to her own movements. Jane stumbled clumsily through the warm-up and seemed as hurried as ever to get through the form. Meanwhile, she continued to remind the class of how tired her legs were from her morning ride (during which she beat all of her riding partners). While she had logged in hundreds of miles on her bicycle, it was obvious that over the course of eight weeks, she had barely learned a thing about Taichi. Jane, however, seemed to think otherwise. It was time, she mentioned in parting, to move on to a "more challenging" endeavor, "now that I have a decent mastery of Taichi."

Reality Check

If people knew how hard I worked to get my mastery, it wouldn't seem so wonderful at all.

—MICHELANGELO

While all of us experience flashes of brilliance and huge leaps of improvement now and again, these flashes and leaps rest on a foundation of piecemeal and often painstaking learning that occurs over a long period of time. Hoping for significant improvement by any other means falls under the label of fantasy. Believing that you have achieved mastery by any other means is called delusion.

Of course, saying that learning takes time does not mean that you cannot improve in a very short period. It is in fact possible to experience improvement in spaces as short as five to fifteen minutes. For improvement to be lasting and deep, however, requires much more time and effort. In the end, we get to choose how lasting and deep we want our learning to go.

After many years of practicing martial arts, I'm supposed to be highly skilled, and in my head, I sometimes believe I that am. Yet, what each additional year of learning gives me is a sense of how little I know and how comparatively shallow my abilities are compared to how impressive I had made them out to be. Perhaps it's because each piece of knowing puts me more in touch with how much more is out there. For even though I've put in thousands of hours of training, I've been clobbered by more than a few who have put in thousands more. And no matter how many thousands of hours I continue to train, two old masters on the other side of the ocean will always be able to toss me through the air with the greatest of ease.

I say this not to discourage you, but rather to expose the vast and joyous expanse of learning that lies ahead of anyone willing to not know the answers and not claim mastery. I notice that whenever I let go of my own need to know more and look superior, it immediately opens the floodgates of learning. No longer needing to defend my "expertise" and "rightness," I feel both relieved and free to explore and discover. Even though not-knowing has a bad name in our culture, it is actually a gift that allows us to stand in wonder. Life, in fact, never really gets boring if you are willing to not know all the answers.

Immersion Learning

Learning intensively seven days a week for a month is not only worth more than doing it once a week for a year, it is much more fun. The more concentrated the learning, the more momentum you gain and the more you find yourself wanting to do it. The more spread out the learning—a little here, a little there—the more backward steps you end up taking while trying to move forward, and less enthusiasm you will feel in practicing. I strongly believe that spreading out learning too thinly is only useful for showing you possibilities for improvement. Immersion learning, on the other hand, leads to dramatic leaps in improvement and allows you to *live* the possibilities.

One of my early immersions, mentioned in the prologue, not only gave me my first real inkling of my learning potential, but allowed me to start living it. Training four to six hours a day, seven days a week brought on enormous changes that I had never imagined possible. By the end of that summer with the masters, not only was my Bagua different, but the way I stood, walked, ran, and simply moved had changed so much that I felt like I had been born into a new body. And the beauty of it was that it was just the beginning: through immersion I had finally found the doorknob.

Obviously, you don't have to train six hours a day, seven days a week to improve—and I generally don't encourage such rigor. To realize significant improvements, however, I do encourage that you make a concentrated effort. For four consecutive weeks, devote forty-five to sixty minutes every day to exploring the lessons. That's equivalent to one long, or two to three short, lessons per day. At most, allow yourself one day off per week from the lessons. If you find yourself overwhelmed after two weeks, take one week off and then resume. I predict that if you concentrate your explorations into two- to four-week time periods, you will be happily surprised by the results. On the other hand, if you start out by thinly spreading out your lessons—doing, for example, one every other week over the next six months—you will probably end up disappointed.

During your immersion, make sure you do at least one lesson from the "Throwing the Ball" series every day (Lessons 1–9). These lessons are an important foundation for running as well as for many other sports. Though the lessons may initially appear simple, paying close attention to the constraints will reveal more and more how bringing awareness to even the smallest parts of your body can increase your power, speed, and agility. Following the constraints in each lesson with ever greater precision will dramatically alter your walking and running over time. As always, it's better to explore with concentrated attention for one minute than to go through the motions and thus pretend to explore while distracted for an hour, or even a lifetime. That one minute equals sixty seconds that you get to move without your habits—move, that is, within the world of learning and discovery.

Finally, keep in mind that it is useful to do a short lesson or even part of a lesson of your choice before your daily run (or your daily walk, if you're taking time off from running). If you're not used to running every day, try adding short runs or long walks on your usual days off.

Sample Four-Week Lesson Plan

What follows is just one of a virtually limitless number of ways to combine the lessons. Some people like to linger on particular lessons, repeating them for a few days or longer. (If this is your style, you may want to spread the completion of all of the desired lessons over a longer period of time—for example, completing the lessons over six to eight weeks instead of four.) Others prefer not to repeat any lessons until going through all of them. Still others choose to skip around at random. There's really no "right" way to approach the lessons, as learning is always an individual affair. Having said this, I recommend using the "Throwing the Ball" lessons as your foundation: begin by working with these lessons more intensively and gradually integrate other lessons.

Week 1

"Throwing the Ball" lessons:

Lesson 1: Posing Questions

Lesson 2: Screwing Foot into Wall

Lesson 3: Flexing/Extending While Throwing

Lesson 4: Stabilizing Your Front Leg While Lying Down

Lesson 5: Flexing/Extending While Throwing in Sitting

Lesson 6: Screwing Foot into Floor

Additional lessons:

Lesson 11: Lift Your Knees (on Your Back, Raising Your Knee toward Your Chest and the Ceiling)

Lesson 13: Behind Your Behind

Lesson 15: Reaching Up

Lesson 27: Where Does My Arm Begin? (Reach and Roll on Your Side)

Week 2

"Throwing the Ball" lessons:

Lesson 1: Posing Questions

Lesson 2: Screwing Foot into Wall

Lesson 3: Flexing/Extending While Throwing

Lesson 5: Flexing/Extending While Throwing in Sitting

Additional lessons:

Lesson 12: Mobilizing Your Rib Cage

Lesson 16: Salsa Hips

Lesson 17: Reach and Roll on Your Back

Lesson 18: Getting Down

Lesson 26: Improving Circulation

Week 3

"Throwing the Ball" lessons:

Lesson 6: Screwing Foot into Floor

Lesson 8: Stabilizing Your Front Leg While Throwing

Lesson 9: Reaching Up While Throwing

Additional lessons:

Lesson 10: Standing Tall Without Trying to Stand Tall

Lesson 14: Water Jugs, Furniture, and Other Things to Carry on Your Head

Lesson 19: Staying Level-Headed

Lesson 20: Making Your Head Lighter

Lesson 21: Walking While Sitting

Lesson 22: Driving Your Knees

Week 4

"Throwing the Ball" Lessons:

Lesson 5: Flexing/Extending While Throwing in Sitting

Lesson 7: Downward Spiral

Lesson 8: Stabilizing Your Front Leg While Throwing

Lesson 9: Reaching Up While Throwing

Additional lessons:

Lesson 17: Reach and Roll on Your Back

Lesson 21: Walking While Sitting

Lesson 22: Driving Your Knees

Lesson 23: Driving Your Knees with a Twist (or Spiral)

Lesson 24: Rodin's Spiral

Lesson 25: Resistance as a Learning Tool

Lesson 26: Improving Circulation

12

Running with
Your Rear End

For every action, there is an equal and opposite reaction.

—NEWTON'S THIRD LAW OF MOTION

After watching runners for several years, I have come to realize that most rely on the power of their calf muscles and hip flexors (the muscles that draw your knee up toward your chest) to propel themselves forward. In either case, what runners normally neglect is the most powerful muscle group in the human body.

Situated in your rear end, gluteal muscles are designed to extend each hip by pulling the thigh backward (see below). Hip extension does two things at once. First, it helps to thrust your whole body forward with a tremendous amount of force.

Second, the backward pulling of one thigh can work in synchrony with the flexion, or forward and upward pushing, of the opposite thigh. This means that the backward motion of one thigh actually helps to drive the forward and upward motion of the other. And this collective action of the two thighs is in large part what gives great runners their "lift" and makes it look as if they are floating effortlessly. The symbiosis, or lack thereof, also explains why many people have difficulty lifting their knees when they run: like me in my track days, they do not understand how to extend their hips while in full stride.

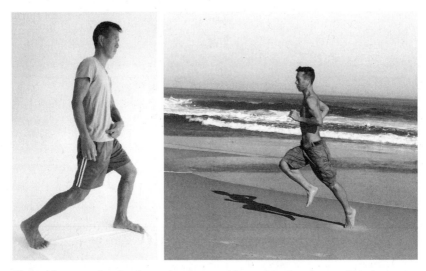

Right: Hip extension, lumbar extension, and thoracic extension working in synchrony. **Left:** Pointing to the anterior superior iliac spine of the pelvis.

Try Lesson 9, "Reaching Up While Throwing," or Lesson 17, "Reach and Roll on Your Back," to get a clearer feeling of how to extend your hips powerfully. When you are finished, go for a short run and notice how each knee travels as you push back with the opposite leg. Are your knees moving higher or farther forward almost by default? Do you feel more power in your stride?

Pushing Off with Your Rear End

To create the above-mentioned "lift" while running requires not just extending one hip while flexing the other, but coordinating the two with the rolling of each foot as it pushes off the ground.

Calf muscles are designed to play an auxiliary, rather than primary, role in pushing off. Specifically, their movement is designed to work symbiotically with your rear end to help mobilize the gluteal muscles. Here's how it works: as you stride forward, the function of your calf muscles is to complement hip extension (the movement that pulls your thigh backward) while they push the ball of your foot downward and backward at the same time. The downward and backward movement of the ball of your foot, in other words, works in coordination with the contraction of your gluteal muscles to pull your thigh backward, and this in turn helps to push your opposite thigh forward and upward with great force. If, for some reason, your calf muscles are not working in coordination with the rest of you, your hips will not extend fully and you will have less driving force, the result of which will be a shorter, more laborious stride.

Obviously, for calf muscles to function in coordination with the rest of you, it is not enough to simply contract them in isolation, but to contract them in synchrony with the flexion-extension (bending-straightening) of your hips and the flexion-extension (bending-straightening) of your knees. Unfortunately, while many people know how to contract their calves, they don't know how to extend their hips and flex their knees in such a manner as to maximize the propulsive force in their stride. The result is that a group of relatively small muscles—namely the soleus and gastrocnemius—end up having to do what they are not designed to do—namely perform the bulk of the work. And when smaller muscles have to take over work for which they are not designed, two things occur: (1) you get far less power because the larger muscles are not fully participating; and (2) the smaller muscles quickly become overworked. Thus, while the gluteal muscles may receive a perennial vacation in such cases, the calf muscles work overtime and consequently become short, tight, and quickly fatigued. Many people complaining of tight calf muscles stretch them frequently to no avail, not realizing that were they to learn how to fully extend their hips and fully bend their knees, their poor calf muscles would be given a chance to rest and function in the way that they were designed to—that is, to play a complementary rather than leading role in the push-off.

You can easily identify "calf pushers" because it looks as if they are shuffling when they are actually trying to run. I myself can identify with such people because this is exactly how I used to run. Obviously I ran this way not because I wanted to shuffle but because I simply knew no other way.

Exploring Lesson 11, "Lift Your Knees," Lesson 13, "Behind Your Behind," and Lesson 17, "Reach and Roll on Your Back," along with the entire "Metatarsals to Metacarpals" series (Lessons 21–26) will help you to gain a much deeper understanding of how to run with your rear end.

Evolution (or God) Doesn't Make Mistakes

In certain parts of the world where individuals travel long distances on foot without the "advantage" of expensive running shoes, and perform daily activities such as eating, socializing, and resting by sitting on their haunches, people tend to maintain a far wider range of motion and more refined sense-abilities than those living in the midst of modern comforts. As a result, the former tend to exhibit superior acture, gait, and stride. While it is not proven, I believe many of the great runners from Kenya, Ethiopia, Morocco, and South Africa owe at least some of their achievement not only to an incredible work ethic but the fact that daily life in these regions often necessitates having greater sense-ability in the movement of everything from head to literal toe.

In contrast, the overwhelming majority of people I've either observed or directly worked with in the United States—including professional dancers and highly trained athletes—tend to exhibit stunted sense-abilities resulting from a modern lifestyle that underutilizes certain muscles in the body. In our culture, one part that appears to be universally neglected is the feet. Specifically, we have stopped using the muscles and tendons that reach from our shins to the tops of our feet and the tops of our toes. I will go as far as to say that in modern U.S. culture, we unconsciously behave as if these muscles and tendons do not exist. Yet evolution (or God) didn't put them there by mistake. Every single muscle is absolutely vital for the full and potent functioning of your entire body. When the above-mentioned muscles atrophy, signaling the extinction of corresponding neural pathways that control them, it can dramatically alter the way you stand, walk, and run.

To illustrate this, I return once again to our first principle of movement (which also happens to be Newton's Third Law of Motion): for every action, there is an equal and opposite reaction. Consider that pushing down into the earth with the ball of your foot requires a certain lifting up of some other part of your foot. What part could that be?

Normally when we push off, we don't use the entire ball of the foot. Certain joints in the ball of your foot (the joints that connect your metatarsals to your toes) normally play a larger role in pushing into the earth as others lift off. In order to push down, there must be a pulling up. And the more forcefully you want to push down with one part, the more forcefully you want to be able to pull up with another. If the muscles that deal with the pulling up have become atrophied, your pushing down will feel murky and less powerful.

Try any of the lessons in the "Throwing the Ball" series (Lessons 1–9) to see how reawakening and reinvigorating the muscles and tendons on the tops of your feet give you more balance, fluidity, and propulsion in walking and running (you'll also notice how it helps you balance in standing). At some point when you have finished the "Throwing the Ball" series, you may choose to explore the "Boxer's Shuffle" series (Lessons 18 and 19), which is a continuation of the sensorimotor concepts introduced in "Throwing the Ball," or the "Metatarsals to Metacarpals" series (Lessons 21–26), which will take you even deeper into sensing how all parts of the feet work can work together with the entire rest of the body.

Each of the lessons in all three series ("Throwing the Ball," "Boxer's Shuffle," and "Metatarsals to Metacarpals") is designed to help you discover the relationship between hip extension and pushing through (or rolling over) the ball of the foot. Some even work with the crucial relationship between hip extension and upper thoracic extension (extension in your upper back). Taken together, the lessons in these series will help you establish a clearer relationship between your feet, hips, spine, shoulders, and even hands. And this mean that by exploring these series, you will begin to experience greater power in your stride while relieving your calves of unnecessary stress and strain. As a side benefit, the lessons will help tremendously in strengthening your feet and ankles, thereby improving your balance while helping to prevent ankle sprains.

Running with Your Upper Body

Hip extension and the tops of our feet are not the only things that we tend to neglect when running. Many overlook the role of the upper body, thinking that it's the legs that should be doing all the work. And your legs really *do* perform all the work yet provide less power when the movement of your upper body isn't properly coordinated with that of your feet, legs, and pelvis. This is because it is impossible to stride powerfully and freely without the full cooperation of your upper body. The thrusting of your rear end and the lifting of your knees must, in other words, occur in complete coordination with not only the swinging of your arms but the rotation, flexion, and extension of different parts of your entire spine. And if your chest, back, arms, shoulders, and neck are not working in coordination with the driving of your knees forward and up (and the simultaneous driving of your metatarsals backward and downward), they end up working against your legs, making them feel both weaker and heavier. The effect is akin to running with a sled tied to your hips.

As I mentioned before, your pelvis acts like the Grand Central Station of force vectors, delivering force in all directions between different parts of your body. Your pelvis, in other words, translates force all the way from your right shoulder down to your left big toe and your left heel all the way up to the top of your head. In this manner, each part of your body has the potential to either cooperate or conflict with parts that aren't directly connected to it. If your upper body is in agreement with what's below your waist, your entire body will be propelled forward with enormous force. But if the two are not cooperating—that is, if you are holding excess tension, or parts of you are not doing their proper share of work (earlier I mentioned that when you don't know how to properly extend your hips, your calf muscles have to take on more work than they are designed for), you end up with internal conflict, and force that would otherwise propel you forward gets dampened. Naturally, you will feel weaker, since you are, in a sense, restraining your own power.

If you watch good runners, you will notice that they are naturally upright and their upper bodies are relaxed. Their stride exudes a certain ease and gracefulness that all of us can emulate when we start to feel how our upper body is able to cooperate with the rest of us. When your arms, shoulders, back, and chest are in sync with your feet, legs, and pelvis, you will have a wonderful feeling of comfort and power throughout your entire body. Your chest will feel like it's floating, and you will subsequently feel tall without trying to make yourself tall. Your elbows will feel like they are pumping automatically, as if by themselves. Your stride will feel smooth and graceful. Lesson 11, "Lift Your Knees," and Lesson 12, "Mobilizing Your Rib Cage," along with the entire "Metatarsals to Metacarpals" series (Lessons 21-26), will help you to integrate the movement of your arms, shoulders, and rib cage with the movement of your legs.

In addition, all of the lessons that involve either stabilizing and elongating your spine or extending and elongating it will give you a sense of how important your upper body is in creating more "lift" and power in your stride. These lessons include:

Lessons 5, 6, 8, 9 from the "Throwing the Ball" series

Lesson 10, "Standing Tall Without Trying to Stand Tall"

Lesson 12, "Mobilizing Your Rib Cage"

Lesson 14, "Water Jugs, Furniture, and Other Things to Carry on Your Head"

Lesson 15, "Reaching Up"

Lesson 17, "Reach and Roll on Your Back"

Lessons 18 and 19 from the "Boxer's Shuffle" series

Lesson 20, "Making Your Head Lighter"

Lessons 22–26 from the "Metatarsals to Metacarpals" series

13

Running with Both Ends

They found that the women could carry 20 percent of their own body weight [on top of their head] with no additional exertion.

—OTTO POHL, "IMPROVING THE WAY HUMANS WALK," *NEW YORK TIMES*

Despite advocating slowing down for the last twelve chapters, I too often feel the pressure to speed up. Hurrying still creeps into my life when my mind gets wrapped up in being somewhere else, doing something else, and thereby prevents me from paying attention to what's in front of my nose. When something feels too challenging, for example, my habit is to either try to get it over with as quickly as possible, or avoid doing it altogether. This used to be my approach to hills—going up them, that is. Of course, hurrying up hills made the experience much less interesting and fruitful because in my haste I failed to realize that the way I was bulldozing through them—rather than lightly bounding up them—actually slowed me down and used up more energy in the process. Furthermore, I lost out on the enjoyment I could have been having—and yes, running up hills can be fun, though your enjoyment will depend on how you do it and whether or not you are forcing yourself.

Several summers ago, while visiting my parents in Southern California, I challenged myself to make a nearby, very steep, and very long hill part of my daily run. After the first day I ended up with very sore Achilles tendons. They were so sore, in fact, that I found myself limping through my run for the rest of the week. I began to worry.

Is this a sign of congenital weakness? Perhaps this is part of the "aging process" that everyone talks about. Maybe I should seek expert advice.

It didn't help that I knew several men my age who had torn an Achilles while playing sports, or that according to a physician friend, doing so is fairly common among middle-age men.

After reexamining how I was running up the hill, I realized that by trying to get it over with, I ended up leaning too far forward and consequently relied too much on my calf muscles. By trying to bulldoze my way through, in other words, I didn't follow my own principle of running with my rear end. Excited that I may have seen through one of my own blind spots, I decided to use the same hill as a playground. What I was looking for was a way to engage my rear end more, and in the process give my calf muscles, and consequently Achilles tendons, a chance to rest.

First off, I had to give up on the idea of covering as much ground as quickly as possible—or more succinctly, getting it over with. By going too fast, I couldn't feel what I was doing, and therefore didn't know what I was doing. Slowing down and being playful allowed me to start to feel what I hadn't felt when I was too hurried. Taking my time to play created space for me to move in nonhabitual ways.

Over the next few days I was delighted to discover much more power in my stride when running uphill. And I was tremendously relieved when the soreness in my Achilles tendons began to subside almost immediately.

Go to Lesson 13, "Behind Your Behind," if you want to discover how much more power you can generate by simply changing your intention as you run uphill.

Discomfort can often be seen as a signpost reminding you that there is a better way. Sometimes it is more a detour than a signpost, as in my case when my Achilles tendons were so tender that I was forced to slow down. My slowing down and subsequent experimentation not only helped my Achilles tendons to heal but allowed me to make new discoveries that in the end allowed me to run faster.

Where Does Your Head Begin?

How you carry your head affects the movement of everything down to your feet. As a result, your head plays an important role in how you use your legs, and thus how much power you gain in your stride. To get a sense of how your feet must adjust to the movement of your head, turn a broom upside down and hold the handle with one hand. Notice how much work you have to do with your hand just to keep the broom from tipping over. Even the smallest movement at the top of the inverted broom requires you to make large adjustments all the way at the bottom, where your hand is.

In order to better understand the connection between the position of your head and how it affects your standing, walking, and running, you first need to feel what's going on. Go to Lesson 14, "Water Jugs, Furniture, and Other Things to Carry on Your Head," if you want a better sense of how even the smallest deviations in how you carry your head affect your posture and thus the way you move.

Running with Your Head

Leaning forward is one of the most popular ways of hurrying when you're on two feet. I've noticed that most people not only lean forward when they walk and run on flat terrain, but they do it when going uphill as well. Many, in fact, lean even more on the uphills. Yet, as mentioned in chapter 8, "Imitation," whether or not leaning works for you depends crucially on exactly how you do it. It is quite common, for instance, to collapse the back of your neck when leaning, and as stated in Lesson 14, "Water Jugs, Furniture, and Other Things to Carry on Your Head," if the back of your neck is collapsing, the center top of your head—what in Bagua is known as your *baihui* point—isn't reaching for the sky. If your *baihui* isn't reaching for the sky, the resultant configuration of your spine will be unsound, perhaps akin to a toppling or collapsing building. Not only is this type of configuration bad for your back and neck, but it saps your entire body of power.

Instead of leaning, I recommend exploring different ways to carry your head. One approach is to rise from the center crown—the previously mentioned *baihui*. Whenever I remember to lift from my *baihui*, it instantly feels as if someone has just added turbocharge to my engine. The feeling of a turbo boost becomes especially pronounced when going uphill. To get a sense of the increase in thrust that can result from how you carry your head, go to Lesson 15, "Reaching Up."

Finally, the relationship between head, neck, and spine brings up the rarely talked about issue of giving your knees enough "room" to lift. Because leaning tends to restrain extension in the hip that is thrusting backward and downward, while at the same time hampering the driving force of the hip and knee that are moving forward and upward, people who bend too far forward may feel like their upper body is getting in the way of their knees. Your spine, in other words, must be sufficiently erect to extend one hip while flexing the other in a manner that maximizes propulsion. This is why, even though sprinters lean way forward in the starting blocks, they do not remain there after the gun has fired. Once they leave the blocks, they quickly come to an upright position, thereby creating more room for their knees to drive both forward and upward.[1] Staying upright and not leaning allows them to generate much more thrust in each stride. Step 5 of Lesson 11, "Lift Your Knees," will give you a clearer sense of how you can lose thrust by leaning too far forward.

---

[1] Michael Johnson and Jesse Owens are two prominent examples of a tall and upright style of sprinting. It is worthy to note that before gaining a world number-one ranking, many people thought Johnson should change his running style. "My coach, Clyde Hart at Baylor, was the only coach while I was being recruited that didn't tell me I would need to change my running style. He never even mentioned it through my college career. And then, once I started my professional career, and then commentators started to say, you know, 'He's got something special. He could be the world record holder if he changes his running style.'" Michael Johnson quoted in Danielle Brennan, "Olympian Michael Johnson on How He Learned to Love His 'Funny' Upright Running Style," *Today*, July 13, 2016.

14

Running with Shoes

Skechers has agreed to pay $40 million to consumers who pur-chased its rocker-bottom shoes under the mistaken belief that the shoes would help give them Kim Kardashian's booty or Joe Mon-tana's stamina.

—RENE LYNCH, "SKECHERS LAW-
SUIT: HOW TO GET YOUR PIECE
OF THE $40-MILLION PAYOUT,"
LOS ANGELES TIMES

Our ancestors did not evolve with hundred-dollar running shoes attached to their feet, and world-class runners like Zola Budd and Sydney Maree didn't use them for most of their formative years. So why do we need them today?

Function and structure reinforce each other in a reciprocal manner. How you walk and run, for example, will determine the wear pattern in the bottom of your shoes. Likewise, the structure of your shoes will largely circumscribe how you walk and run. So when you impose on your feet the structure of, say, a new pair of running shoes, it will affect the functioning of your entire body. The support from your shoes, for example, forces your entire body to adjust while at the same time limiting the mobility of the myriad joints in your feet and ankles. The padding in your shoes serves to displace shock and consequently acts as a substitute for how you would otherwise use the muscles and tendons surrounding the joints in your feet, ankles, knees, pelvis and spine to redirect the incoming force. The elevation in the heels of the shoes serves to tilt your body forward as if you were standing on a hillside facing away from the hill. As your nervous system gets accustomed to standing on this artificial slope, all of the muscles from your heels to the base of your skull shorten and remain short in response. Most of us don't notice the shortening except in rare instances when we try to touch our toes, sit on our haunches (that is, squat with our heels still touching the floor), or do a somersault. What we more likely notice, however, is the tightness and fatigue in our calf muscles, or perhaps how uncomfortable our lower backs feel.

Shoes are to your feet what earplugs are to your hearing: while both protect you, that protection also serves to insulate your sense-abilities from the outside world. Generally speaking, shoes tend to limit the range of motion in your joints, and muffle the sensory input that would otherwise register below your knees. Here, it's important to note that your muscles, tendons, and joint surfaces do not exist in isolation. They are, in fact, attached to your nervous system and cannot function without it. So when you begin to limit the variety of choices for your muscles and tendons, you are also limiting the amount of movement patterns available to your brain. A simplistic view of it goes as follows: where unused muscles and tendons gradually become stiff and weak, neural pathways that once governed the varied movement of these muscles and tendons begin to die off. And as neural pathways die off, sense-ability atrophies and movement patterns begin to disappear from your repertoire. For many people, the result is having not only weaker but clumsier feet and ankles, which in turn translates to a weaker stride.

Strengthening Your Feet
and Ankles *Sense-ably*

The possible effect of well-supported shoes does not, of course, mean that you cannot be a good or even great runner if you wear them.[1] As you have surely noticed, virtually all of today's runners, including the world's best, are sporting the latest "technological advances" in footwear. The likelihood of developing weaker feet, a less powerful stride, and self-destructive movement habits, however, is much higher in a culture such as ours, which encourages everyone not only to wear shoes but to wear highly supported ones, with an elevated heel, from an early age. Compared to people who grow up wearing no shoes, or only the flimsiest of footwear, we not only have weaker and more rigid feet and ankles but walk and run with less stability and power. Thus for us shoe-wearers, it is particularly useful to find ways to strengthen our feet and mobilize joints down below that have become stiff and inflexible over the years.

Finally, if we accept the previously stated theme that the movement of one part of your body affects the movement of all other parts (see chapter 10, "Following Instructions: Where Do My Knees Begin?"), we can understand that changing the way you use your feet will alter the way you use your entire body—all the way to the top of your head.

Take note that what you've just read is not an exhortation to throw out your running shoes and go run a marathon in bare feet or in flimsy sneakers. Doing so could result in injury because your body has already become not

---

[1] For people with loose ligaments, well-supported shoes can even enhance the stability in their feet in ways that their own muscles are not yet able to (I insert "yet" here because it is possible for these people to gradually learn to use their muscles to create that stability). In such cases having a good deal of support may actually be beneficial by conferring added stability where none previously existed.

only accustomed to having a great deal of support but dependent on it. The muscles and tendons in your feet and legs, for example, lack the strength and flexibility to deal with losing this support. Your entire spine has become accustomed to a more limited range of motion that is part and parcel to wearing shoes.[2] Obviously, it would be a shock to your entire system—muscles, tendons, ligaments, and mind—because you cannot in one split second magically acquire the sense-ability necessary to adapt to such startling new conditions. Since years of wearing shoes have led to your current state, it will take at least a little time for your feet, spine, and nervous system to regain some of the independence they probably once had in early childhood.

If you want to experiment with wearing less support or none at all, I recommend you start off by doing it for short periods. You can, for example, try walking for short distances in an old pair of Converse All-Stars. If you are willing to spend a little more money, you can test out a pair of so-called "barefoot" shoes that have virtually no support and thus allow for a much fuller range of motion in your feet, ankles, knees, hips, and spine. And if you don't want to spend money, yet still desire a sense of how humans walked and ran for aeons, you can, of course, try going without any shoes at all.

Take note that in all my suggestions, you are encouraged to initially walk, not run. Once you have become accustomed to walking with less support, you can experiment with running very short distances—maybe a few steps at a time to start with—and working your way up to fifty meters at a time. As long as you are gradual in building up distance, you will maximize improvement while minimizing the risk of injury.

The lessons in the "Throwing the Ball" series (Lessons 1–9) are among my favorites for helping students gain better awareness of how their feet, and even toes, relate to the rest of their body. Each of the lessons works very effectively in awakening and strengthening not only your feet, ankles,

---

[2] Your entire spine needs to adjust to standing, walking, and running in bare feet. If it does not make the proper adjustments—and it won't simply do so without a period of learning—your feet will strike the ground with a resounding thud, sending shockwaves all the way up to your head.

and lower legs but your thighs and gluteal region as well. As a side benefit from doing the lessons, the greater control in your legs, along with increased rotational force in your hips and spine, will likely improve your performance in other sports and even daily activities. And whether or not you engage in other sports, you will nonetheless feel a marked difference in the way you stand and walk in the short time it takes to do just one lesson.

Everything Below Something
Is a Foundation for That Something

A tough surface inside the shoes of athletes can help protect their feet, knees, and ankles, according to a new study that involved 17 members of the Australian woman's soccer team.

—JOHN O'NEIL, "VITAL SIGNS: PROTEC-
TION; TEXTURED INSOLES WIN HIGH
SCORES," *NEW YORK TIMES*

As mentioned in chapter 5, "Intention," our first principle of move-ment—"for every action, there is an equal and opposite reaction"—ensures that everything in your body works in a reciprocal fashion. Everything on top affects everything on the bottom and vice versa. You could say that something below something else acts like a foundation for that something else. Thus, your feet act as a foundation for your ankles and your ankles for your knees. Weakness in any of the foundations will cause a chain reaction all the way up to the top of your head. Since your shoes form the final foun-dation between you and the ground, it is important that they form a secure base. If either shoe tilts even the smallest amount to the right or left, for example, everything above it must adjust. Believe it or not, even your other foot and leg will be affected. Any unevenness in either shoe, in other words, requires your entire body to compensate, which could translate to overus-ing certain muscles while underusing others. And the consequent muscle imbalances can, over time, lead to uneven wear and tear in your joints.

Your movement habits involve a multitude of factors, including the way each foot lands and rolls or pushes off, and all the intricacies that make this happen, from how your ankle joints articulate, to the contraction of your hamstrings, to whether your head is cocked a fraction of an inch to one side. Too much uneven wear in your shoes and you will start to exaggerate these habits, reinforcing movement patterns that may be inefficient and possibly damaging in the long run. This is perhaps most obvious in people who have collapsed arches. If you look at the shoes of somebody with flat feet, you will likely see that the wear and compression patterns in the tread and sole reinforce their particular way of grinding their ankles and knees. The effect doesn't stop there, but actually continues up to the hips, pelvis, spinal cord, and eventually, the head.[3]

Of course, most of us do not produce such extreme wear patterns on our shoes. We do have our own characteristic ways of wearing out shoes, however, that if gone unchecked will reinforce any imbalances we may already exhibit, or even create ones where none had previously existed. In light of this, I urge you to examine how you feel during and after a run, considering that wear patterns can contribute to discomfort as well as decreases in power.

I encourage you to play around with different types of shoes and take your time getting used to whatever it is you put on your feet. Take everything as an experiment—one in which, by exploring movement slowly, you are creating

---

[3] It is important to note here that in the vast majority of cases, fallen arches have much more to do with muted sense-abilities and unhealthy movement habits acquired in early childhood than genetics. I strongly believe that it is possible to improve the strength and flexibility of your arches by learning new ways to use your feet, ankles, and indeed, entire body. Considering that flat feet are a symptom of atrophied muscles and lowered sense-ability, learning could be an effective way to literally raise the arches. Both the "Throwing the Ball" series (Lessons 1–9) as well as the "Metatarsals to Metacarpals" series (Lessons 21–26) can be very effective in improving the strength and pliability of your feet. Exploring these lessons can, over an extended period time, begin to strengthen your arches if they are weak or fallen. I have seen my own previously low arches grow significantly since I began experimenting with the way I use my feet. That said, these lessons alone are not sufficient to rectify all types of imbalances and weaknesses that might be afflicting your feet. There is a myriad of movements and positions available in the Feldenkrais catalogue of lessons as well as in various martial arts, forms of dance, styles of yoga, and "natural movement" regimes that could be equally or even more helpful.

new neural pathways that simultaneously lead to increased balance and a more powerful stride. Try, for example, walking around without your insoles and see what happens. Experiment with insoles that have nodules or construct your own to see how the added sensory information alters your gait and stride. Spend five minutes in shoes with a lot of padding and notice how it affects your posture, gait, and stride compared to five minutes in shoes with little to no padding, such as racing flats. Take a few backward or sideways steps in super-slow motion—as if doing Taichi—and see how this feels in bare feet compared to when wearing shoes.[4] Whatever style of shoe you play with and whatever movements you make, notice if you feel more or less of the ground as a result. See if you have more or less control over your feet and legs. Notice if your joints feel more or less comfortable. Sense how seemingly minor changes actually affect the way your feet land and push off. If you try shoes with less support, or walk for longer periods in bare feet, you will be employing muscles and tendons that haven't been used in a long time. Your feet may initially tire more quickly as a result, but they will continue to get stronger as long as you don't push yourself too much. And this brings me to the most important point: be gentle with yourself, and don't turn play into a chore, or you will risk injury. Consider that changing shoes is simply an option, not a necessity. You may in fact love your current style of footwear and never want to change.

Lesson 16, "Salsa Hips," will help you discover how a supple rib cage improves smoothness and power in both your gait and stride. This is a particularly useful lesson if you are transitioning to shoes with less padding, or even considering joining the barefoot running movement.

---

[4] Every time you change what's on your feet, your nervous system has to readjust itself. The less accustomed you are to whatever you are wearing, the more time it will take to adjust. I notice a huge difference in the way my foot strikes the ground and the way my upper body wants to move whenever switching from my usual pair of worn sneakers to a new pair, or a different style of sneakers with less of a sole, or to dress shoes, which tend to have higher heels, more padding, and less flexibility in the sole. Dress shoes normally make me feel clunky at first, while my feet, legs, and spine are finding ways to accommodate the new foundation under my feet. In contrast, shoes that have minimal padding and more flexibility in the sole give me a tremendous boost in my push-off as well as a great deal more maneuverability. In either case, however, I am continuously listening to my ankles, knees, pelvis, and spine so that they can adjust to the change.

PART 3   MORE LIFE

(Skip this part if you are still in a hurry.)

15

Compulsion

I am always against "no pain, no gain." Because pain is always the body rejecting whatever you are doing. It's your body telling you, "I don't want to do it; it's not right for me." But people can force themselves to do it, sometimes because they come from a hard life, and have had to work so hard just to survive. That becomes the mentality, therefore anything you do must become hard, uncomfortable. That is not a good thing.

—FONG HA, 5TH GENERATION YANG-STYLE TAICHI MASTER

Like many newcomers to Feldenkrais, I expected instant results. Most people come seeking help with injuries and pain. I came because when I read Moshe Feldenkrais's book on compulsion, I knew he was talking about me.

It was the second week of my Professional Feldenkrais Training and our director, Frank Wildman, was leading us through another series of what were supposed to be gentle movements on the floor. After five minutes, my neck started to hurt. Yet, through gritted teeth, I persevered.

Ten minutes later and still following Frank's instructions, my neck hurt worse. If I'm doing everything right, why does it hurt so much? When Frank walked by, I flagged him down.

"My neck hurts," I said helplessly, as if expecting him to wave a magic wand and instantly make the pain disappear. Frank stopped in his tracks and looked directly at me. "Stop," he said, then turned and walked away.[1]

The one thing I didn't consider.

Looking back now, I realize how hard I was trying to be a good student. I felt compelled to follow every instruction to a T lest I miss out, or look bad in Frank's or someone else's eyes. Today it seems totally comical that I was ready to tear my head off its moorings for the sake of following instructions. In reality, both my misinterpretation of the instructions and the need to "just do it" not only resulted in pain but prevented me from learning. Rather than tuning into my senses, I was on autopilot, trying to "get it over with."

Stress, Anxiety, and Perception

After teaching for many years, I've noticed that losing one's senses is a common coping strategy. The process is akin to working on an assembly line where you put together gadgets as they pass by on a conveyor belt. At slow speeds, the work is manageable. But what happens when the conveyor belt starts to go faster? You have to go faster to keep up, and at some point your level of anxiety will increase very quickly. Meanwhile your ability to sense and feel will decrease proportionally, and your work will get sloppier and sloppier. Ironically, because your perception is decreasing to a pinpoint, you won't notice the button in front of your face that says, "Push to stop the conveyor belt." And you won't hear the voice over the loudspeakers saying, "This is all a game. Please don't take it too seriously."

Inability to deal with stress leads to anxiety, which in turn mutes perception—the vital tool for dealing with stress. So generally speaking, the more

---

[1] Apparently, "stop" is a phrase commonly issued not only by Bagua masters but Feldenkrais Trainers as well.

pressure you feel, the higher your anxiety level; the higher your anxiety, the less you can sense and feel; the less you sense and feel, the less you are capable of dealing well with stress. It is a vicious cycle.

Considering that much of modern life has become some version of gadgets whizzing by on a conveyor belt, it should be no surprise that most of us are in a terrific hurry. It is a surprise to many, however, that hurrying makes us less competent to deal with the conveyor belt.

Another Way

Many people don't enjoy running as much as they could because they do it in ways that aren't so pleasurable. On top of that, many force themselves to do it when they really don't want to. Yet, what if there were ways to train that gave you more pleasure, and you just hadn't discovered them yet? And what if, unbelievably, some of these training methods translated to running exactly the way you wanted to, when you wanted to? Wouldn't you then be delighted whenever it came time to go for a run? Naturally, if you associated running with lightness, freedom, breathing fresh outdoor air, or a challenge that you were up to (rather than one that overwhelmed you), then running would become something you were always eager to do.

If you look at children running around on the playground, you won't see grim expressions on their faces (compare children's expressions to the ones you see on the faces of most adults). How do children do it? Do they ever look at adults and wonder how so many of us have managed to turn what could be play into drudgery?

Unlike children, we don't do what we want. Specifically, whereas we tend to want results and ignore the process, children care less about results and fully live the process. And in doing so, they allow themselves to move in any manner they like, sometimes trotting, sometimes skipping, sometimes hopping or jumping or rolling on the ground or spinning in circles or stopping or chasing each other or doing cartwheels or kicking their own bottoms as they move about. Is it any wonder they find so much pleasure in running?

The All-or-Nothing Approach

We don't do what we want because we don't actually know what we want. And we don't know what we want because most of us have been forcing ourselves to do what we don't want for so long that we have come to see the world as black or white, all or nothing, either I run five miles or I don't run at all. If we want to start enjoying running more, we have to stop forcing ourselves and begin looking between the all and the nothing.

At this point you may be thinking, if I don't force myself, I won't do it. Yes, this is a possibility, but only because most of us haven't made distinctions between different ways to run. Most of us have been attending the ever more hurried assembly line of modern life for so long that our perception has become severely narrowed. As a result, we tend to look at running—and indeed, the rest of life—as a choice of all or nothing. You can observe such narrowing every day when, for example, somebody from the Midwest says, "People from LA are aggressive drivers," or someone from LA says, "People from the Midwest are too slow." Implicit in each statement is the grouping of all people from LA or the Midwest being one way or another. Similarly, when we make running a grim reality of life that we need to do to get in shape, feel good about ourselves, improve circulation, have friends, attract a mate, or something else, we are unconsciously deciding that all types of running are grim.

In other words, by assuming that our approach to running is the only way, we are unwittingly neglecting every other way to do it. We are ignoring the fact that between the all and the nothing, there is actually a lot of something.

How to Get Yourself off the Couch

"But what about times when you can't get yourself off the couch?" you might be asking. "Wouldn't you be better off forcing yourself?"

Here again, we have an all-or-nothing situation. There are many ways to get off the couch. The ones most often used are on the compulsive side of will-power. But there are many other ways that involve the loving side of willpower.

One of the reasons we have trouble getting ourselves off the couch to begin with has to do with our compulsive all-or-nothing conditioning.

Who wouldn't want to sit on the couch watching TV if the other alternative is to suffer through another bout of self-torture? In this case, you are sensible not to get off the couch.

Most of the exercise and training programs I have witnessed or personally experienced (some of which I designed myself) have to do with either whipping yourself into condition, or more likely, having someone else do the whipping for you. You'll notice that gym memberships peak right after the New Year when everybody's made a resolution to get in shape and lose weight, but attendance plummets shortly after the first month. Is it because people are lazy?

Maybe. Or maybe it's because people are sensible. That is, they are still senseable enough to know that lashes on the back are generally no good for you, even if you happen to be the one holding the whip. Of course, this is not to say that pushing yourself, being coached, and having discipline are intrinsically bad—in fact, both the prologue and chapter 11, "There Are No Shortcuts, No Secrets, No Magic Pills," address the positive side of discipline. Rather, what I am saying is that most of us require much less, if indeed any, prodding or coercion to get off the couch. Few exercise and running programs, nevertheless, start at a manageable pace for the individual. They are highly generalized to zip people into shape as fast as possible with little or no regard to learning or fundamentally improving stride, coordination, balance, and agility. Obviously, starting this quickly is going to require a good deal of prodding. Considering the number of dropouts, however, starting this quickly is not the best way for everyone.

Even if I am highly disciplined and willing to be my own drill sergeant, I will run into strict physical and emotional limitations. Though I may get in shape and improve rapidly at first, my improvement will still be limited by my resistance to the pushing. Overcoming resistance doesn't mean that either the resistance itself or the attendant faulty mechanical habits have magically disappeared. Unless I allow myself to slow down and tune into my senses, both will continue to weigh down on my stride, preventing me from becoming nearly as fast and powerful as I could be. Moreover, the pressure I put on myself will likely lead me to associate running with suffering. As a result, I may never truly enjoy the activity and unwittingly find myself wanting to avoid it. And when I actually succeed in avoiding it—taking a day off, for example—I may feel defeated and unworthy.

Leading with Desire Versus Pushing with Compulsion

As I mentioned above, people embarking on a new training regimen often find themselves in over their heads. Because their initial exposure to running may have been too strenuous, they may have unconsciously stereotyped the activity to be something that requires a high tolerance for pain and suffering. In this regard, I recommend that workouts not be overwhelming lest they inspire fear and loathing in the person performing them. In high school, I myself feared "hard days" precisely because I had been overwhelmed by previous experiences. Even when training on my own, I often set the bar too high, believing if I didn't run fast enough and far enough, the workout wasn't any good. Training like this too often was very effective in taking all the joy out of running, though not so effective in making me want to get off the couch. Indeed, during the summers when I trained alone, I would procrastinate all day and put off my runs until the evening.

This attitude stands in sharp contrast to my experience with tennis and basketball—two sports I took up after quitting track and triathloning. Rather than drearily looking ahead toward my next engagement, I would be brimming with eagerness and excitement. The very thought of playing either sport would send my heart leaping. You'll notice that people engaging in a sport that they love never identify that particular sport with dreariness (and if they do, it is likely because they are turning play into drudgery by focusing too much on extrinsic rewards). Yet people who love their sport run enormous amounts on the court—often to the extent that they find themselves gasping for air. They do all this willingly and out of desire, not compulsion.

For those who do not respond well to being pushed—and I believe this is most of us—what we need is to be led in a way that allows us to bring the love back into running. Like children who slow down or walk when they are tired but on the other hand rarely need to be encouraged to run, we need to listen to our senses. In this manner we will rediscover our own pacing and increase our distance and workout intensity in a manner that suits our individual desires.[2]

---

[2] If you are near the ocean, try the "Chasing Waves" game at the end of chapter 6, "Have You Lost Your Senses?," or make up your own game where your attention is on something other than burning calories or putting in miles.

Rediscovering Your Own (Ever-Changing) Pace

Do not depend on the hope of results. When you are doing the sort of work you have taken on ... you may have to face the fact that your work will be apparently worthless and even achieve no result at all, if not perhaps results opposite to what you expect. As you get used to this idea you start more and more to concentrate not on the results but on the value, the rightness, the truth of the work itself.

—THOMAS MERTON

After you've gotten into the groove of running in a more playful and exploratory manner, you may be tempted to count your miles or the amount of time you spend on each run. You may want to set a bar like *x* number of miles today, or *y* number of minutes tomorrow. If you feel so inclined, I recommend you do it, but only as an experiment. What we are testing is whether setting the bar increases or decreases your enthusiasm for running. Try it once and see what happens. If the bar makes you want to avoid running, then lower it or simply remove it altogether. If it makes you more enthusiastic, then continue using it or even consider raising it. Again, be experimental in the process.

From my personal experience, counting miles was somewhat self-defeating because I tended set the bar too high, as in the habit of most people trying too hard to succeed. In doing so, it made me not want to run, and when I was running, it made me wish the miles were over and done with. I may have done better to set the bar much lower or not to have one to begin with. Some of my teammates, on the other hand, preferred to plan out how many miles they would run every day, and for them it seemed to encourage and excite them rather than take the joy out of the activity as it did for me. Whatever the case may be for you, listen to your desire. It will guide you to the right place.

As a final note on pacing, consider *fartlek*, the Swedish "innovation" on running that gained mass popularity in the 1980s. *Fartlek*, which means "speed play," is for me simply a derivation of what children do naturally: add variation—whether in pacing or type of movement. Varying the pace and type of movement you perform can allow you to tune into what your body really wants. It means giving yourself the option of slowing down, speeding up, or even stopping and walking at any given moment. Be playful and add other styles of movement such as skipping, doing somersaults, kicking your own bottom, jumping small shrubs, going backward, sideways, or in circles, or even dodging imaginary obstacles. Basically, you are allowed to do anything you want, and by granting yourself this freedom, you are likely to discover new ways to do your running—or perhaps more accurately, to be your running. As a result you will avoid the kind of slogging through runs that I experienced in my days of competing. Take note of how you feel after doing (being) your own style of "speed play," which could well include "slow play." I recommend you keep a journal just for such observations. You will be surprised to discover that in the process of observing yourself as such, you will get to know yourself better, and the positive effects of self-knowledge will ripple into the rest of your life.

16

Fear

In our muscles as much as in our ideas, we are trapped by the tyranny of what we come to regard as "normal."

—DEANE JUHAN, *JOB'S BODY*

"Move your legs! Move, damn it!"

Joseph Del Real was a loving and ultimately demanding "old-school" coach in the narrow sweat-filled basement gym where I was attempting to learn some basic fundamentals of kickboxing. He seemed as frustrated with my sudden and seemingly total loss of coordination as I was shocked about it. It was as if, the instant the bell rang, my body suddenly forgot how to move.

The funny thing is I couldn't have followed Joe's simple instructions to save my life—though ironically, it felt like I was indeed trying to save my life. In real time, I was hardly even conscious of his frantic yelling. It wasn't that I didn't want to listen, but that nothing, except my opponent's fists, seemed to penetrate my skull during those terrifying two-minute rounds inside the boxing ring. As a totally inexperienced middleweight, trying to avoid the Goliath fists of a heavyweight who outweighed me by a hundred pounds meant an instantaneous loss of all my sense-abilities. It was as if all controls in the proverbial cockpit had suddenly been jammed. From a neurophysiological standpoint, I was in the grips of the startle reflex.

The Startle Reflex

We enter the world with one reflex fully intact. It is called the startle reflex and consists of two phases. In phase 1, muscles that straighten your arms, pull your head back, and lift your chest suddenly contract with tremendous force. These muscles are called extensors because they extend your body and pull your body wide open like a starfish. A split second after the start of phase 1, phase 2 begins with the violent contraction of all your flexors—the muscles that pull your body in the opposite direction: inward, in the direction of a tight ball. The startle reflex, comprising not only your response to, but your experience of, fear, gears you up for either fight or flight. Fear through the startle reflex is a necessary response in the face of real danger, and it has allowed our species to survive on the planet. Without fear there would be no human race. With it, however, the human race may be driving itself to extinction.

The startle reflex is itself neutral—that is, neither intrinsically good nor inherently bad—and simply a necessary tool bred into the mammalian nervous system to maximize chances for survival. How we use it or get used by it, however, can determine what kind of lives we lead, and even what kind of society we create. The more triggers that we bind to the startle reflex, the more fearful and anxious we become as individuals. Unfortunately, in a fast-paced society run by high-strung individuals, people will tend to associate more and more of the world with fear and anxiety—the latter simply being the fear that things are not going to work out. As a result, things that are not even remotely life-threatening will on some level be perceived as such. Getting stuck behind a slow-moving car, for example, often triggers a distinct physiological response, which is based on some (mostly unconscious) level of the fear of being late or perhaps missing out on something important. Being late or missing out are not in and of themselves life-threatening, but our hypervigilance, clamped jaws, constricted breathing, and clenched fingers belie a certain fearfulness that says a hungry lion is ready to pounce. On some deep unconscious level, we are afraid of our own demise when the clock is ticking and the traffic light turns red.

Lions, Tigers, and Bears

Most adults in modern society exhibit some degree of chronic hypervigilance. This means that we are unconsciously stuck in a mild to serious state of fight or flight—our responses to everyday life becoming a habitual reenactment of some portion of the startle reflex, more commonly known as anxiety. And this chronic reenactment bespeaks an attitude of certainty: we are certain on some (mostly unconscious) level that our life is under constant threat.

When I carry anxiety into the world, I am responding to life as if it were something to be survived. Yet when my life is not truly being threatened, to merely survive is to disrupt my ability to sense and feel. Fear, no matter how small and seemingly inconsequential, is always linked to some increase in muscular tension and consequently some decrease in control. If I carry anxiety into everyday life—meaning that anxiety has become a habit—all of the physiological changes in my body along with the concomitant narrowing of my perception will become the baseline for what I consider to be normal. While this state of dis-ease will color every movement I make, I will remain largely unaware that it could be any other way. I will not realize, in other words, that someone placed sandbags on my shoulders, and that that someone is me.

Such dysfunctional coping has to do with the fact that the same adaptability of the nervous system that allows me to acquire greater sense-ability and thereby produce more fluid and powerful movement also allows me to lose my senses and inadvertently sabotage my movement. Thus, if I carry anxiety for a prolonged period, my nervous system will forget the feeling of freer, more coordinated, and powerful movement. And in no longer being able to sense and feel it, I will be unable to replicate it. Recall that being able to move in certain ways means being able to sense and feel how to move in those ways. The less I am able to sense and feel myself, in other words, the less coordinated I become.

The result of all of this is a state of normalcy that feels heavy, ungainly, and deadening. In this state of what philosopher and somatic pioneer Thomas Hanna calls "sensory amnesia," the attendant muscular constriction affects all of my movements, thereby requiring more effort to perform even simple tasks such as sitting, standing, and walking. As a result, I will feel a certain heaviness as I go through my days and may even begin to feel helpless or cursed. At some point, I may look to surgeons, God, bad genes, or some other outside source to bear the responsibility for my plight.

Anxiety: Certainty About Uncertainty

If anxiety is part of my everyday existence, it could mean that I have on some level stereotyped a large portion of life, seeing it through all-or-nothing lenses. The "all" in this case is in the persistence of the anxiety, which I generally carry with me, and which could be manifest as dread, or more likely in a gnawing feeling that something is not going to work out.

From a movement perspective, stereotyping itself is simply the extinguishing of movement possibilities through the exclusion of a wider array of movement patterns. While this exclusion is most often connected with fear, it is also fundamentally rooted in moving too fast to notice the something between the all and the nothing—or in this case the sometimes between the always and never. Not everything is immediately life-threatening—not even red lights, angry bosses, complaining spouses, or surly people at the checkout counter. Unconsciously, however, our stereotyped reactions often make us respond as if they were.

Chronic tension and anxiety in the absence of something life-threatening is, in other words, a form of certainty about the world. It is a certainty that the world is on some level dangerous. And while this is sometimes true, often it is not. The world is, in fact never static, but rather constantly fluctuating and uncertain. Yet if I take a fearful, anxiety-ridden posture into the world, I am behaving as if the world were static, and in this case, statically dangerous.

Looking at it this way, chronic anxiety is a posture that goes hand in hand with my fear of uncertainty. Because it is chronic, and therefore largely fixed, the attitude beneath my fear could be one of certainty that uncertainty is bad and consequently to be avoided. And masking my fear with aggression, arrogance, chauvinism, feigned positivity, or some other form of suppression does not necessarily make me suffer less (though in some cases, it may temporarily delay the suffering). Rather, it simply adds a clause to my largely unconscious worldview: The world is dangerous and I can beat it—with intimidation, condescension, complacency, duplicity, denial, or some other form of blocking. In the latter case, I have simply overlain one parasitic posture on top of another, resulting in two constricted postures vying for position within one body.

Having Anxiety Means You're Human

I have met countless people of great compassion and sensitivity, people who would describe themselves as "conscious" or "spiritual," who have battled with CFS, depression, thyroid deficiency, and so on. These are people who have come to a transition point in their lives where they become physically incapable of living the old life in the old world. That is because, in fact, the world presented to us as normal and acceptable is anything but. It is a monstrosity.

—CHARLES EISENSTEIN

Though one could easily conclude from what I've written above that to show any sign of anxiety is to reveal some degree of moral weakness (and to show no signs is to indicate, therefore, moral superiority), I prefer to take a more integrated view on the matter. As I mentioned in chapter 9, notes 3 and 4, *all* feelings and emotions are part of what make humans human. Even though suppressing particular feelings and emotions could give off the impression of being happier, more positive, more inspired, more stoic, more agreeable, or even more suitable for a desired job opening, doing so over the long term could lead to feeling degraded, dehumanized, and perhaps more like a machine than a human.

From this perspective, both the feeling of fear, anger, anxiety, indignation, or any other "negative emotion"[1] and the expression of any of these could bear just as much legitimacy as the feeling and expression of "positive emotions."[2] And this means rather than rejecting that which makes us human, we might do better to acknowledge and accept it. For only by doing so do we have the opportunity to discover more benign and constructive

---

[1] For the sake of simplicity I am conflating feelings and emotions, though from a neurophysiological standpoint, they are distinctly different. For more on the subject see, Manuela Lenzen, "Feeling Our Emotions," *Scientific American Mind,* April 14–15, 2005. For an in depth study, see Antonio Damasio, *The Feeling of What Happens: Body and Emotion in the Making of Consciousness* (Boston: Mariner Books, 2000).

[2] And in an age of growing precarity (where wealth continues to be siphoned from the pockets of working people to the bank accounts of the wealthy), living with some level of anxiety, sadness, indignation, and even anger seems to me to be quite normal. A good deal of work has recently emerged regarding the legitimacy of so-called "negative emotions" and how they are a normal and very human response to a dysfunctional culture and political economy. Philosopher Charles Eisenstein states: "Back in the 1970s, dissidents in the Soviet Union were often hospitalized in mental institutions and given drugs similar to the ones used to treat depression today. The reasoning was that you had to be insane to be unhappy in the Socialist Workers' Utopia. When the people treating depression receive status and prestige from the very system that their patients are unhappy with, they are unlikely to affirm the basic validity of the patient's withdrawal from life. 'The system has to be sound—after all, it validates my professional status—therefore the problem must be with you.'" See Charles Eisenstein, "Mutiny of the Soul," *Reality Sandwich,* October 7, 2008. Like Eisenstein, journalist Johann Hari sheds light on how our current political economy influences and, in some cases, drives both depression and addiction. For a fascinating read, see Hari's *Lost Connections: Uncovering the Real Causes of Depression—and the Unexpected Solutions* (New York: Bloomsbury, 2018) and *Chasing the Scream: The First and Last Days of the War on Drugs* (New York: Bloomsbury, 2015). Looking at employment in general and service-oriented forms in particular, sociologists Arlie Hochschild, Louwanda Evans, and Jennifer Pierce look at how the commodification of emotions tends to have a dehumanizing effect. For an in-depth look, see Arlie Russell Hochschild, *The Managed Heart: Commercialization of Human Feeling* (Berkeley, CA: University of California Press, 2012). For a quick look into the matter, see Adia Harvey Wingfield, "How 'Service With a Smile' Takes a Toll on Women," *The Atlantic,* January 26, 2016.

ways of dealing with our emotions and thereby gain a deeper awareness of both ourselves and the myriad factors that affect us.[3]

---

[3] Writing on the anniversary of the Christchurch massacre—yet another racist act of terrorism inspired in part by the same reality TV star and favored candidate of the Christian Right who, since being elected to the White House, has inspired so many other hate crimes—I feel compelled to emphasize the importance of not only searching for more benign and constructive ways to deal with our thoughts, feelings, and emotions but understanding that doing so may not be enough to rescue us from the evil in others, or that which dwells within ourselves. The obvious reason for this is because while you might be meditating, practicing yoga, getting therapy, or attending self-help seminars as a way to deal with your stress, I could be spray-painting swastikas on the walls of the local mosque or synagogue to deal with mine. Yet, even assuming you and I both choose the same culturally accepted approach to deal with our respective problems, most of those available, whether quasi-spiritual, religious, psychological, psychiatric and pharmacologic, or somatic, will tend to focus solely on the individual to the virtual exclusion of examining the sociological and political-economic strings by which that individual is tethered to society. And this means that most of the solutions offered, while providing possible succor for our respective wounds, will likely fail to address many of their direct and indirect causes. Furthermore, divorced as such from examining the organizing structures of society, this type of *non*-integrated approach consequently runs the risk of making us better suited to fit into society while at the same time ignoring the possibility of making a society better suited to humanistic ideals. (Obviously not a huge problem, unless, of course, our society happens to be one that tolerates, and in some cases even promotes, rising levels of inequality; rising levels of poverty; grossly unequal access to health care; rising levels of student debt; drug profiteering; war profiteering; illegal invasions of sovereign nations; mass incarceration; impending sea level rise and increases in catastrophic weather events [as the inevitable result of our failure to sufficiently address human-induced climate change]; widespread sexism, racism, xenophobia, and homophobia; voter suppression; police brutality; racial profiling; persecution and exploitation of undocumented workers; widespread homelessness; summary detention [incarceration] and deportation of refugees; prosecution of people who attempt to rescue or otherwise aid refugees; mass surveillance; suspension of right to habeas corpus; state-sponsored terrorism; state-sponsored torture; corporate bailouts; global environmental degradation; and genocide.) With all of this in mind, perhaps a more integrated, humanistic, and even effective approach to dealing with the human condition would be to examine the individual *within* the context of society and political economy—a radical, though not necessarily popular, or even new, idea that goes at least as far back as the moment Jesus turned over the tables of the moneylenders (and actually much farther back, if you consider debt forgiveness to be an integral part of both Mosaic Law and Sumerian edict). For a fascinating account of the history of debt forgiveness going back to the third millennium BCE, see Michael Hudson, *And Forgive Them Their Debts: Lending, Foreclosure and Redemption from Bronze Age Finance to the Jubilee Year* (Dresden, Germany: ISLET, 2018).

ACTURE, FEELINGS, AND EMOTIONS

To experience how the complex interplay of assumptions, judgment, and emotions play a crucial role in affecting acture or posture, try the following experiment:

Stand up, or simply sit at the edge of your chair so that your spine is relatively erect. Notice how you are breathing? Which parts of you expand more? Which parts feel heavier or more constricted? How long does the back of your neck feel?

Imagine being in a public space and noticing somebody standing in the corner of the room looking at you. Can you sense how this changes your breathing and posture? If you are very attentive, you will notice changes throughout your entire body.

What if the person looked at you disapprovingly? Notice how much more this changes your breathing and acture.

What if you discovered that the person isn't looking at you, but is actually blind? Can you feel how your breathing suddenly expands again and how much lighter you feel?[4]

---

[4] Note that the initial class, gender, race, age, sexual orientation, body type, political affiliation, or any other attribute that our imagination conjures up plays a crucial role in our visceral response and reveals our unconscious assumptions and biases. As I mentioned earlier, assumptions and biases are neither intrinsically bad nor intrinsically good, but as long as they remain unconscious and we consequently remain unaware of their effect on us, we will be limited to our habitual response, which will be more or less malignant or benign, depending on the circumstances and personal values of all parties involved.

17

Certainty

I think if we ever reach the point where we think we thoroughly understand who we are and where we came from, we will have failed.

—CARL SAGAN

Our dominant culture is one of being certain. People under its sway (this would be virtually everyone) sometimes recoil at the mere suggestion that there is another way, not realizing that other possibilities exist outside of the one way they have chosen.

I am no exception.

All of us experience absolute certainty when we're sure we're right. During these times our body language, facial expressions, and words all confirm that we already have all the answers. I call it the "I know! I know!" attitude, and what it is really expressing is that uncertainty should be avoided.[1] "I know! I know!" is the compulsive side of certainty that protects our rightness about the world, and thereby makes us feel safe and secure. In the process of locking out the world, however, such absolute "knowing" can prevent new sensations and feelings, and thus ideas and insights, from entering.

---

[1] In a teacher, it might show up as the "What do you mean you don't get it?" attitude.

Everybody falls into this trap some of the time. The problem is that many of us fall into it most of the time. Our perception narrows accordingly, and the potential for learning all but disappears. Like the captain of the *Titanic,* we assume that our way is the best and perhaps only way, so we continue barging full steam ahead toward that "harmless" piece of ice.

Certainty and Perception

In general, certainty keeps me safe and my life relatively stable. It helps me categorize the world such that I know that all apples are red and shiny, and drinking coffee at dusk will keep me up all night. In this manner, certainty guides me through daily life without having to think too much and shuttles me toward things I like and away from things I don't like, and which may even be dangerous. Thus, I will happily jump into an expensive car knowing how comfortable the ride will be, but avoid jumping in front of one as it speeds past because I am certain that doing so would lead to injury or death.

There are times, however, when certainty puts us or others at risk. I may be certain, for example, that driving on the right side of the road is a good idea. Yet if I happen to be in Tokyo instead of Los Angeles, my certainty will likely lead to an accident. I may be certain that the man waving his gun and running toward me is going to shoot me. But what if the man running toward me is actually trying to catch a bus, and his gun upon closer inspection turns out to be a newspaper? This would be problematic if I were a police officer and had already drawn or even fired my weapon.

In all cases, too much certainty is often the major factor in limiting my perception. I literally see, hear, taste, smell, and otherwise sense less of what is actually around me when I am too certain. This is because what I see, hear, taste, smell, and otherwise sense is strongly colored by what I expect to see, hear, taste, smell, and sense. If, for example, apples are supposed to be shiny and red, I may never notice the green ones, which my mind will have unwittingly placed into the "not apple" category.

The Necessity of Certainty

You could say that certainty begins at birth in the form of the startle reflex: if startled, all newborns will automatically respond with absolute certainty in the manner described earlier. Yet to thrive in the world, our newborn will eventually need to know more than simply how to contract himself into a ball. This is why he is naturally curious and begins exploring the world as soon as he enters it. And as he explores the world, he is simultaneously exploring himself.

As our newborn explores, his mind arranges crude sense-abilities into finer ones. Simple and crude movement patterns thereby become more precise ones. The sum of all of these patterns will eventually become his certain ways of moving and expressing himself. Each level of refinement can be seen as a milestone—a new level of mastery and therefore certainty upon which he can construct ever more refined and complex movements. Once satisfied with crawling, for instance, he will work toward standing and eventually walking.

From this perspective, you could say that certainty is an organized database that keeps our growing infant from having to relearn the same things over and over again. In this regard certainty allows our newborn to gather, organize, and reorganize material. His growing database, which contains emotional, intellectual, and movement-based components, forms the foundation upon which he learns new ways to emote, think, and move. His growing database acts, in other words, as a foundation upon which he learns new movement patterns and therefore new behaviors, the collective sum of which could be considered the expression of his being.

The Necessity of Uncertainty: Exploring Versus Performing

In the animal kingdom, all action falls under either one of two categories: (1) uncertain, exploratory movement, which is the process of sharpening sense-abilities and thereby learning new movement patterns; or (2) certain,

performatory movement, which is the process of utilizing (but not improving) existing sense-abilities, to make use of already mastered skills and
acquired movement patterns.

Both exploratory and performatory movements are necessary for survival—the former allowing us to learn, and the latter giving us a way to
sidestep learning so that we can perform necessary and independence-
giving functions such as walking, talking, putting on clothes, or bringing
food to our mouths. In our early years, most of our actions will naturally be
of an exploratory nature since we begin life with only crude sense-abilities
and therefore virtually no movement patterns in place other than inborn
reflexes.

As we get older and continue honing our sense-abilities, we simultaneously acquire more movement patterns and thereby gain more independence. When this occurs, performatory movements begin to take greater
precedence. By the time we reach adolescence, our movement repertoire will
have become so expansive that exploration itself, while still beneficial,
will become largely unnecessary. By this point, in other words, most of us will
have mastered such an enormous amount of skills that we can navigate daily
life without having to learn anything fundamentally new. Perhaps this is
why, for many middle school students, everyday life will become less about
learning and more about repeating old patterns.

Given this, adolescence could be thought of as the phase during which
certainty and habit surge in their influence over executive functions while
uncertainty and exploration begin their steep descent into what in many
cases will turn out to be permanent hibernation. Put more simply, adolescence is when most of us begin to settle into ways of moving and expressing ourselves that we will likely carry into adulthood and perhaps even
to the grave. And even though it is considered a time of great freedom
and experimentation, the experimenting itself—whether with athletics,
art, music, drugs, sex, or ideas—often occurs within the confines of basic
patterns learned in childhood. Thus, from the perspective of both behavior
and learning, adolescence is for many, a time when we begin to live life
the way we lived it yesterday. And this means that by the time most of us
have settled down into our careers and partnered life, we will have already

spent several years doing things the way we have always done them—that is, using the same movement and therefore behavioral habits that we likely acquired in our youth.

The Power of Uncertainty

Being creative means being able to relax into uncertainty and confusion.

—FRITJOF CAPRA

Obviously, there is nothing wrong with doing things the way we have always done them if the way we have always done them works. The problem is that it often doesn't, at least not to the degree that we would like—which brings to light the fact that exploration, while unnecessary after a certain age, remains highly useful if we want to continue learning and improving. Exploration is unnecessary, in other words, if we want to continue living the way we are living, but highly useful if we want to learn how to live more fully.

Great athletes, martial artists, and dancers are to some degree certain about their movements, but not so certain that they stop exploring and adding new patterns to their "movement database." So even though their movements are efficient, powerful, and precise beyond most people's comprehension, they continue to seek a higher level of mastery. They are, on some level, uncertain. This is why they are masters.

To test your level of "mastery," go to Lesson 17, "Reach and Roll on Your Back," and try it again. After finishing, continue to the next paragraph.

The Line Between Learning and Getting It Over With

When you attempted the last exploration in Lesson 17, where did you put your foot? After observing hundreds of students over the years, I discovered that nine out of ten move their foot on a line that is parallel to their midline.

It's so uncanny that it's as if I had given the instruction: "Move your foot on a line that is parallel to your midline." That, however, is not the instruction. It's also not not the instruction. What it is is an interpretation of the instruction.

The actual instruction simply asks you to try five different locations for your foot. Any five. If your reaction is to move toward and away from your buttock in a line parallel to your midline, you are missing out on a vast number of possibilities. Why? Because rather than confining yourself to a line (fig. 1), you can move your foot in an area (fig. 2).

Moving your foot down a line when you could move it in any direction is needlessly restricting your movement. You can compare it to painting a line straight down the length of a tennis court and then attempting to play a match without stepping off the line. Doing so might be a fun experiment if it is your intention to see what happens under this constraint. But what if every time you played you only stayed on the line, forgetting that you were allowed to step off of it? Without even realizing it, you would be making the game much more difficult and wondering why your opponents always trounced you. You might resign yourself to being a bad tennis player with little hope of improving. You might never realize that your real opponent is not the person across the net.

At some time in the future you may choose to go back to Lesson 17 and try it again. If you haven't done so already, see to it that you begin to explore putting your foot off to the side a little. You can even put it in places that you think are outlandish. Be playful about it and in the process of being playful, you will make many discoveries. You will begin to discover foot placements that give you more power to roll your hip. Surprisingly, even discovering less than optimal places for your foot will contribute tremendously to your learning.

As a final note, I think of facing uncertainty as opening the door for new possibilities to emerge. We may not always welcome uncertainty (I rarely do), and we may face it with some level of trepidation (I almost always do), but simply facing the unknown often creates openings where none previously existed.

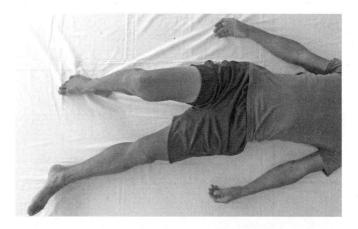

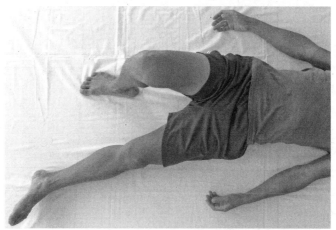

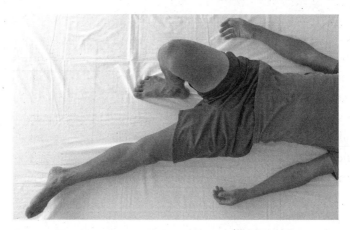

Figure 1. The foot moves downward in a straight line.

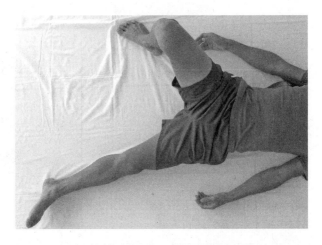

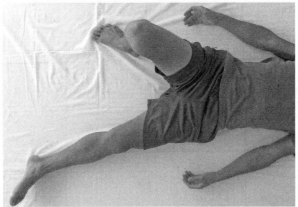

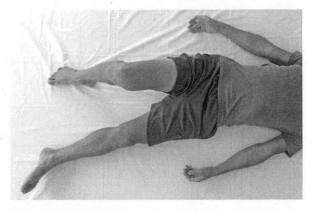

Figure 2. The foot covers a wider area—you have the freedom to move your foot anywhere.

Epilogue:
The Rest of Your Life

(Definitely skip this part if you haven't slowed down yet.)

> *When you are wholehearted about something ... when you are where you want to be and are participating fully in the moment you are in—sometimes enthusiastic, sometimes mellow—you will experience a new sense of aliveness. You will experience a surge of energy, renewed vigor. This is not because there is actually an increase in energy, but because you are not constricting it quite so much.*
>
> —ERICH SCHIFFMANN, *YOGA: THE SPIRIT AND PRACTICE OF MOVING INTO STILLNESS*

Over twenty years since my introduction to Feldenkrais and martial arts, I find myself ever more experimental with and intrigued by movement. When I think about how much better I feel in middle age than I did in the supposed prime of my life—during which I was too busy hurrying to be interested in paying attention and exploring—I know that slowing down has fundamentally altered my being. It's not just that I move with much more awareness than when I was younger, but moreover that I perceive more of myself and therefore more of life now that I tune into my senses.

Contrary to my experience in school and organized sports—both of which tended to encourage mimicry, imitation, and rote—Feldenkrais, Bagua, and Taichi led me to tune in and come to my senses. The crucial element of slowing down to enhance sense-ability has reintroduced curiosity, wonder, and learning into my life, and subsequently turned my bodymind into an exciting laboratory through which I am continuously making important discoveries. After one of my early immersion periods into Bagua and Feldenkrais, for example, I began to experience the joy of walking for the first time. Where walking, like everything else in my life, had once been a chore to be gotten over with, it had suddenly become a process to be enjoyed through entirely new sense-abilities—ones that made my gait light, fluid, and powerful. Walking for miles through the streets of New York City after having just returned from my first summer with Master Ge and Master Li, I remember feeling vibrant and playful, like a child who has just been given a new toy.

By the end of my second summer with the masters, I was stronger, faster, and more grounded than ever, even though I didn't lift weights and hadn't run a step in ten years. Bagua and Feldenkrais were helping me develop a deeper connection with my own body, far beyond anything I had ever experienced during my days of competitive racing. Confident that it would show in my running, I jumped into a 10K road race as an afterthought and placed third in my age group—one that seemed to include an inordinate number of balding fathers who were apparently in the habit of eating too many dinner rolls. Though placing well among overweight middle-aged dads wasn't exactly earth-shattering, what astonished me was the fact that my stride felt much freer and more powerful than it did when, well over a decade prior, I was running five to ten miles a day. This feeling would become more obvious weeks later while visiting a friend in Toronto.

When I arrived at my friend's house, situated in an old Slavic section of the city, we decided to walk down the street to a neighborhood restaurant. Two years of immersion learning had resulted in my gait becoming fluid and smooth, while my chest felt as if it were floating upward, rather than weighing me down as it had for most of my life. My head was literally higher and my gaze less downward than just a couple of years earlier—not because I was trying to hold everything up, but because through all the exploring I had done, my skull had naturally gravitated to a new, more comfortable position. The ease and comfort I felt, a natural result of more deeply sensing myself, allowed me to take in more of my environment. In contrast to much of the way I had been surviving most of my life by unconsciously tuning out of it, I felt much more at peace and tuned in to everything around me. I can still remember the redbrick row houses, the overcast sky at dusk, the brightly lit health food store that we stopped at on the way, and the sound of what could have been Polish spoken by two elderly women as they strolled past us.

Perhaps the only thing I wasn't tuned into was where I had left my wallet. Upon reaching the restaurant, I realized that I had forgotten it back at the house. Knowing that my friend wouldn't mind waiting the few minutes it would take for me to make the round trip, I turned around and began striding back in an easy and relaxed manner. The funny thing is that no longer in a hurry (or for that matter, trying to beat out the nearest overweight middle-aged dad), I felt faster and lighter than ever. In fact, my stride felt so effortless and strangely powerful that it was as if I were gliding on air. Right then and there, for the first time in my life, I had a real sense of how great runners must feel as they glide down the track. By this, I don't mean that I had suddenly reached an Olympic caliber, but rather that I could finally relate to the effortless power I had witnessed in so many great runners. Try as I had during my track days, I could never come close to imitating the runners that I so admired. I couldn't imitate them because I had never slowed down enough to accurately sense what I was doing, and consequently had no sense of what they were doing. During these moments of effortless striding, however, I felt at long last like I was in on their secret. And it took not trying to run fast to really notice how fast I had become.

As I continued easily down the street, I knew I was finally not only on the road to being a better runner, but on one to freedom. Over ten years removed from running and without the slightest interest in returning to competition, I had become faster than I ever imagined was possible. The unmistakable feeling of power and freedom had finally arrived because I had finally stopped trying to be.

"Side" Benefits

For those of you who have made time to explore the lessons in this book, you may have discovered over the course of weeks or months that along with running better, other aspects of your life have started to change. For example, you may have noticed positive changes in your acture—which, perhaps, you no longer think of as posture—improvements in your ability to perform other sports, and greater ease in performing everyday activities such as walking, mowing the lawn, or even doing the dishes.

How could all of this be possible just from having slowed down?

Your nervous system is remarkable in its ability to integrate deepened sense-ability into all of your movements so that even though you may have set out to improve your running, other movements have improved as well. This is why performing other activities may have become more interesting and even pleasurable. Your sleep may have become deeper and more restful as your increased sense-ability has decreased residual tension, thereby allowing your chest cavity and abdomen to become more expansive and your back and shoulders to let go. You may gradually become more aware of how you move through your days and be able to feel subtler tensions in your body well before they build up into something like a backache, headache, or sore shoulders. You may find yourself more able to let go.

Holding On to Life Is
Not the Same as Living It

A chronic muscular contraction is not something that somebody else is doing to me. It is something that I am doing to myself.

—STANLEY KELEMAN, *YOUR BODY SPEAKS ITS MIND*

Letting go can be scary. Holding on feels comparatively safe. Perhaps there is something biological about it: grasping is one of the first natural reflexes that a newborn infant displays. She holds on firmly to her mother.

Yet growing up means letting go of mom and many other things. We must periodically let go because holding in itself prevents us from grasping anything new.

People and objects are not the only things that we hold onto. Holding is also written into our habitual movement patterns, and these patterns constrain to a large degree how we deal with life. With this in consideration, it is of enormous benefit to acquire new movement patterns that give us more freedom in how we choose to encounter and move through the world—patterns that allow us to let go of stress rather than cling to it.

If, for example, in the process of slow exploration I learn ways of breathing and moving about that are less restrictive and less laden with tension, I will be starting from a calmer and more confident place to begin with. I might, for example, begin to literally feel how particular parts of my rib cage are able to move and expand, allowing more breath to flow through me. I may notice a softening in the deep muscles of my lower belly that not only releases tension, but allows for a greater exchange of gasses and fluids through my tissues and internal organs. I might discover ways to move my spine that relieve the muscles in my shoulders and the back of my neck. Embodying these new movement patterns, I will begin to move, and therefore respond differently, possibly facing the world with less anxiety and fear.

Dealing with life's downs, however, is not the only or most important benefit of letting go. For life is not only about coping with the unexpected, the unpleasant, and the tragic. It is also about feeling pleasure, joy, and wonder. Consider that excessive holding has a twofold effect: it makes me more anxious and fearful in times of increased stress, and it makes me less able to feel pleasure, peace, and joy in times when I am not faced with difficulties.

We can only become aware of pleasure and feelings like joy and peace through our senses. If we totally lacked sense-ability, pain and fear would no longer dog us. But then again, pleasure and love would not exist. Looking at it this way, pain and fear are not evils to be extinguished, but a necessary part of life to be dealt with sensibly. By being able to sense and feel more, you do just that: create the possibility for a sense-able rather than sense-less response. Moreover, you simultaneously allow yourself to truly experience pleasure and joy. Improving your sense-ability, then, not only allows you to better deal with stress, but it gives you the opportunity to more fully experience what it means to be alive.

When "Normal" Means Abnormal

The "normal" life that most humans lead is a life of unconscious self-destruction. If they were conscious of it, they would not do this to themselves, but as it is, they have no choice. They are hapless victims of a society in which a regular and insupportable burden of stress is consciously accepted as normal while, unconsciously, the central nervous system is brutalized to the point that it can no longer sustain the burden.

—THOMAS HANNA

As we saw in chapter 7, "To Be or Not To Be," movement and response-ability are both colored by sense-ability: the less I can sense and feel myself, the fewer options I will have in both responding to the world and express-ing that response. Hurrying and forcing, for example, express themselves through the constriction of muscles in my spine, rib cage, abdomen, and pelvis such that my breathing automatically becomes shallower. Hurrying as a habit consequently leads my normal state to be one of constriction and reduced oxygenation, not because I consciously choose it, but because my mind has forgotten how to let go of and expand all of the tissue surrounding my lungs. Thus, if I compulsively hurry and force my way through daily life, I will over time literally lose the sense of what it feels like not to hurry and force. Through habituation, in other words, the neural pathways that allow for a fuller movement of my entire rib cage, spine, and pelvic basin will have been pruned away. As a result, I will have fewer resources for staying calm, more likely acting with some measure of anxiety and frustration when faced with stress. In the extreme, I may even withdraw or explode under the mild-est of adverse conditions. Whether I close down timidly, strike out angrily, or simply clench my jaw and bear it, I will feel stuck with the situation, not realizing that what I am really stuck with is a limited number of ways of both perceiving and expressing myself.

Stress can be a powerful learning tool if, rather than looking at the stressor in isolation, we examine our response to it. From this perspective, stress can be seen as something that we inadvertently accumulate when we don't know how to release it from our bodies and minds. Thus, how I react to whatever new befalls me depends crucially on how much stress I have accumulated to begin with. If, for example, I am typically a shallow breather, or tend to grip hard on the steering wheel, or suck my belly in tightly, or clench my jaw, I will not have at my easy disposal deeper ways of breathing or moving about my world that would allow me to handle any added stress with a measure of calm. And the crux here is not simply that I deal poorly with added stress, but that I am already stressed-out to begin with—even before the outside world intervenes. The sense-abilities that I'm habitually locked into, in other words, are ones that keep my normal level of tension and discomfort at a higher level.

The irony here is that my normal everyday state undermines my own well-being. I do not maintain such "normalcy" to intentionally harm myself or those around me, but rather as a matter of habit and familiarity. Significant here is the fact that not only are certain muscles perpetually clenching and holding on, but that the mind to which they are attached is telling them to do so. It is as if I am saying to myself, "Hold on, or else!"

Or Else What?

A bit of advice

given to a young Native American

at the time of his initiation:

As you go the way of life,

you will see a great chasm.

Jump.

It is not as wide as you think.

—JOSEPH CAMPBELL

"Or else what?" is a question that cannot easily be answered. And perhaps this is why it is so common in our culture to live with fear and certainty. We are certain that the unknown is something to be avoided, so we hold on to what is familiar. But holding on is not really living. And were it possible, knowing the unknown before it arrived would make life rather uninteresting.

Life is uncertain, and by trying to evade uncertainty, we are evading life. Perhaps this is why clinging to certainty can be so disruptive to our ability to feel pleasure. For we cannot extinguish pain from our lives without simultaneously extinguishing pleasure. We cannot anaesthetize ourselves with painkillers, video games, TV, or the latest gadget and at the same time feel more deeply.[1] Sensing more in our bodies and our hearts requires that we turn down the volume of extraneous inputs so that we can begin to notice the whispers of wind blowing, allow new sensations to enter our bodies, hear the voices deep within ourselves.

At the extreme, certainty imprisons us like royalty high up in our castles (or, if you prefer, politicians in the Capitol) and prevents us from truly seeing and knowing others. Safely behind our moat, we can view maps of the world, look at photographs of it, or even watch TV programs that simulate it. Yet from this distance we are not really part of the map-making, or the picture-taking, or indeed, the living. Our certainty, in other words, which resides in our thoughts, sets us apart from the world, which rests in our bodies through our sensing and feeling. As our sense-abilities consequently shrivel, we lose touch with the world itself. Rather than experiencing life directly, we filter it through our "I know! I know!" attitude, trading compassion and understanding for defensiveness, wonder for being right, living for surviving.

Perhaps the greatest loss in this process of desensitization is the fact that we have turned against ourselves. Certainty in the form of "shoulds" and "shouldn'ts," otherwise known as self-judgment, limits our ways of moving,

---

[1] There are, of course, exceptions to my generalization about video games being anaesthetizing. For some interesting descriptions of the possible positive effects of gaming, I recommend Edward Snowden's memoir, *Permanent Record* (New York: Henry Holt & Co., 2019).

behaving, and expressing ourselves. We become a stereotype of ourselves rather than being ourselves. For it is precisely because we think we know ourselves that we are no longer in touch with our sensing and feeling—or in other words, who we really are. Because we are not good enough, we try to be something that we are not. Rather than being, we turn to not being.

We have, in other words, become human not beings living within highly regulated modes of thought and behavior that are circumscribed by perpetual certainty, otherwise known as the all-or-nothing, otherwise known as fear.

What are we afraid of?

The answer is right in front of our noses: we are struggling so hard to not be because we are in fact afraid of being. And we are afraid because the act of being, which is simply sensing and feeling more deeply and therefore living life more fully, carries no guarantees.

Not Quite Living

Many of us exert a great deal of effort trying to get the present moment out of the way. Whether the moment involves driving to work, work itself, exercising, spending time with a loved-one or friend, eating, or even having sex, we are often not quite here, but rather trying to get to the next moment before the present one is fully felt in our bodies. Indeed, we rarely experience the present because we are racing so quickly toward the future. And we are racing because we are mired in the past, believing that what befalls us in the present has already been experienced before. Our certainty about the present moment has become a sort of "been there, done that" attitude slavishly driving us toward something less predictable and more stimulating—something, in a word, new.

Boredom, which has become epidemic in modern society, must be conquered with the newest video games (notice how anything more than a few years old is no longer worth playing), TV, the internet, snacking, amusement parks, or other forms of non-interactive, passive entertainment. Chronic pain, which has become so widespread as to become a medical condition in and of itself rather than just a symptom, must be quickly subdued with drugs. Deep-felt pleasure, which is so absent as to have entire industries devoted to simulating it, has come to be replaced by cheap imitations (which are actually quite expensive when you think about it) that assault our taste buds, overstimulate our glands, dull our minds and eventually leave us in despair. What we want is for life to be more stimulating, pleasurable, and exciting and therefore less predictable, painful, and boring. What we get is the opposite: more predictability, pain, and boredom.

The irony in all this is that nothing about life is predictable or boring—except, that is, when we are not present to experience the something between the all and the nothing. By trying to make life less predictable, painful, and boring, however, we simply do the opposite. Perhaps herein lies the message that life is giving us: we cannot improve life by avoiding it; we cannot infuse life with what we think is more life and not end up subduing it.

Sense-ability and Freedom

There was a group of students who would occasionally bring Professor flowers to see him practice his love of flower arranging. I have no sense of how good he was at it; his arrangements were beautiful, but the formal art of flower arranging is beyond my understanding. I was always awed, though, watching a man of his great power displaying utter delicacy as he trimmed and shaped his floral arrangements. His delicacy resonated in that gentle place in me that I had blocked off for my adult life because I feared it wasn't manly. One of the many gifts he gave me was the way he led me back to the best part of myself.

—WOLFE LOWENTHAL, *THERE ARE
NO SECRETS: PROFESSOR CHENG
MAN-CH'ING AND HIS TAI CHI CHUAN*

Sensing and feeling are the filters through which life enters. By choosing how much we are willing to sense and feel, we are actually choosing how much of life to let in at any given moment. Life simply is, and moment-to-moment we are determining what fraction of it gets in.

In the end, what increasing sense-ability lends us is greater discerning power over what we let in and what we don't. We literally have more choices and therefore more freedom when we are able to sense more of the something between the all-or-nothing. Increasing sense-ability, in other words, allows us to more precisely determine what is at each moment so that we have more choice in the matter. Decreasing sense-ability, on the other hand, blocks out more of what is so that we have less choice. Of course, this doesn't mean we should never block things out, but rather that most of our blocking is actually unconscious and thus limiting. I may consciously choose to put in earplugs before attending a rock concert, for example, but (unconsciously) forget that they are in after leaving the concert. By putting in the earplugs, I am exercising choice. By forgetting that they are in, however, I am losing the choice of hearing my surroundings.

Unconscious habits are where we remain deaf to what is because we have forgotten to take out the earplugs. If, for example, I can't clearly feel how my rib cage moves with each step I take, I am not only deaf to certain movements in my own body, but unaware of how to use the movements in order to generate more power. Unable to clearly sense my own movements, in other words, I automatically move with less control over, and hence less power in, my stride. I may think I am free, yet if I ignore the option of improving my sense-ability, the only remaining option is to try harder in order to improve.

Here is where I am faced with a critical choice: I can act with certainty by hurrying up and trying harder, or I can slow down and simply allow myself to be. In the former case, I reduce my sense-ability, increase my "deafness," and consequently reinforce my habitual movement patterns. In the latter, I take out the proverbial earplugs, increase my "hearing," and move outside the realm of habit.

In this sense, running faster is a choice, though not the one most people believe it to be.

But getting myself to run faster is not why I began slowing down. And getting you to run faster is not why I wrote this book.

Postscript

A Final Word (or Ten Thousand) on Running

*[In the] "humanistic conception," with its roots in the Enlight-
enment ... education is not to be viewed as something like filling
a vessel with water, but rather, assisting a flower to grow in its
own way ... in other words, providing circumstances in which
the normal creative patterns will flourish.*

—NOAM CHOMSKY, *CHOMSKY ON MISEDUCATION*

We begin at birth to explore many of the basic sensorimotor patterns necessary for survival, independence, and performing complex actions such
as running. In this sense, the moment we are born, we begin learning to
run. This latter process continues all the way until the age of seven, which
is roughly the point at which each of us arrives at a more fully mature and
adult-like manner of walking.[1] Beyond that, our gait, and therefore our

---

[1] Most children exhibit what scientists call "mature gait" around the age of three. Their
manner of walking, however, will continue to develop, more closely resembling that
of an adult only in the ensuing years. "The gait of a seven-year-old child has the same
differences from an adult's gait as a three-year-old's does—but to a lesser degree. Adult
cadence, step length, and velocity cannot be achieved until adequate growth occurs.
Duration of single-limb stance in a seven-year-old is about 38 percent. (In adults,
duration is about 39 percent)." Mary Keen, "Early Development and Attainment of
Normal Mature Gait," *Journal of Prosthetics and Orthotics*, 5:2 (April 1993), 37/25.

stride, will not undergo any major changes unless we happen to engage in the type of sensorimotor learning that is capable of systematically altering our basic movement patterns.[2] For adolescents and adults, this means the way we run has been essentially determined by what we did many years ago—by the movements and thus sensorimotor patterns we did and did not explore in early childhood. For those among us who are not exemplary runners (almost all of us), this means that our running stride exhibits the same sensorimotor, and thus exploratory, deficits that were evident in childhood. And for the select few who are so fortunate, it means the explorations and types of movement we engaged in after early childhood have made up for some of these deficits, thereby allowing our stride to come a little closer to the ideal.

Ideal Stride

Ideal stride falls within the domain of ideal image, which is a vital, albeit mostly unconscious, driving force behind every exploratory movement.[3] For given the enormous degrees of freedom available in the human body and the innumerable ways those degrees can be combined, every movement we make, from the more primitive, such as sitting at a piano and pounding the keys with one's fists, to the more complex, such as sitting at the same piano and playing Rachmaninoff's Piano Concerto No. 3 in D minor to a sold-out crowd in Carnegie Hall, can be performed in a more or less

---

[2] Just as some of the most sensorimotor patterns, such as lifting one's head and rolling over from supine to prone (and from prone to supine), serve as the foundation for learning to stand and eventually walk, walking gait serves as the foundation for running stride. Put more simply, and to use an old cliché, you can't run until you've learned to walk.

[3] Exploratory movements in particular and exploration in general are necessary for learning. In contradistinction to exploratory movements, those of a performatory nature are undertaken with a specific goal in mind, whether it happens to be crossing the finish line in an 800-meter track race in front of everyone else, doing a pirouette with supreme artistry and emotional content, or simply reaching down to the floor to pick up a piece of paper.

ideal manner.[4] Anything that involves movement, including every form of music, class of sport, form of dance, type of martial art, and style of acrobatics, adheres to its own ideal image, or as the case may be, various related and sometimes even conflicting ideal images. Ideal images unique to any movement-based discipline are in fact what allow us to differentiate it from all other movement-based disciplines.[5]

More broadly speaking, every person both consciously learns and unconsciously generates ideal images that help to classify, identify, and organize the entities, events, processes, theories, conceptual frameworks, and phenomena that are part of their particular world.[6] Given the myriad differences in how any two people consciously conceive of or unconsciously perceive (or don't perceive) any given entity, event, process, theory, conceptual framework, or phenomenon, it is important to note that an ideal image

---

[4] The range of possibility increases by orders of magnitude when we consider that, primitive reflexes aside, every movement we make is coordinated by a highly evolved and complex brain. According to neuroscientist Vilayanur S. Ramachandran, "The human brain is made up of about 100 billion nerve cells, or neurons. Neurons 'talk' to each other through threadlike fibers that alternately resemble dense, twiggy thickets (dendrites) and long, sinuous transmission cables (axons). Each neuron makes from one to ten thousand connections with other neurons. These points of contact, called synapses, are where information gets shared between neurons. Each synapse can be excitatory or inhibitory, and at any given moment be on or off. With all these permutations, the number of brain states is staggeringly vast; in fact, it easily exceeds the number of elementary particles in the known universe." V. S. Ramachandran, *The Tell-Tale Brain: A Neuroscientist's Quest for What Makes Us Human* (New York: W. W. Norton, 2011), 14.

[5] A world without ideal images is, in fact, an undifferentiated world—one therefore devoid not only of sport, dance, art, and science but concepts and distinctions. One could go as far as to say that ideal images emerge from nature itself via the vehicle of natural selection. To be more specific, the origin of any given species could be thought of as the origin of the ideal range of genetic expression—one, in other words, that maximizes the potential for survival and reproduction under the given circumstances.

[6] Note that the concept of ideal image I am using throughout this postscript corresponds to the following linguistic concepts: "typical case prototypes," "ideal case prototypes," and "essential prototypes." For some nice examples of each, see George Lakoff, *Moral Politics: What Conservatives Know That Liberals Don't* (Chicago: University of Chicago Press, 1996).

is always exclusive to some degree or another, depending on how it is (very often unconsciously) constructed. To be more inclusive, an ideal image must remain more vague and general. Conversely, to be less inclusive, it must become more precise and specific. This is why the general ideal image of, say, an airplane might include having a cockpit, fixed wings, and an engine, without specifying exactly what components are used for the cockpit, wings, and engine. Once we start getting more particular and specify, for example, a single-seat cockpit, laminar flow airfoil, and a Rolls-Royce Merlin engine, the ideal image obviously narrows, thereby becoming more specific and less inclusive.[7]

It follows that general ideals normally remain steadfast for long periods until some groundbreaking influence such as a major discovery, newly introduced perspective, or cultural revolution (and thus, political-economic revolution) alters our conception of the entity, event, process, conceptual framework, or phenomenon under scrutiny. Ideal images for airplanes, for example, stayed relatively stable after the concept of fixed wings with separate systems for lift, propulsion, and control gained popularity, even if technological improvements led to specific changes.

In contrast, highly specific ideal images often depend on short-lived, quickly changing, and quickly forgotten events such as incremental technological advances (for example, in microprocessor design for computers), fashion trends ("What kind of jeans are in style this year?"), pop-culture trends ("What recording artist sold the most records last year?"), design trends ("iPhone 6, versus iPhone SE, versus iPhone 7"), or the results of head-to-head competition ("Who is this year's Eurovision winner?"). Thus, where the aforementioned ideal image of an airplane has for over a century generally included fixed wings and separate systems for lift, propulsion, and control, the changes in specific details of the fixed wings and systems for lift, propulsion, and control (as a result of technological improvements and design changes) have led to both specific changes in, and greater variation of, what is considered ideal.

---

[7] This description narrows the ideal down to a specific make and model known as the P-51 Mustang.

Ideal Image: General Versus Specific

Given the enormous variation within the general population with regard to sensorimotor awareness and thus sensorimotor control, our ideal images for human movement are always exclusive to some degree or another. As with our relationship to any entity, event, process, theory, conceptual framework, or phenomenon, the more general the ideal image for a particular move-ment or movement sequence, the more inclusive it will be. Conversely, the more specific the ideal image, the less inclusive it will be. Virtually all adults, for example, run in the same general manner, even if each of us will exhibit specific differences that mark our uniqueness in the world. In this case, the "general manner" in which all adults supposedly run must be defined broadly enough to include virtually all adult styles, if the statement is to be true. If we narrow the boundaries of our ideal image, we could also say that all world-class runners run in the same general manner even if each one exhibits her own characteristic stride. In this case, "general manner" is only in reference to world-class runners, a subset of the set of all adults, so that the range of specific characteristics of the ideal image is much narrower. Thus, "general manner" in the second case means something quite differ-ent than it did in the first because world-class runners share some specific attributes with other world-class runners that they don't share with non-world-class runners.

Of course, there are also specific attributes that a world-class runner doesn't share with anybody, including other world-class runners. So even though world-class runners are in many respects similar enough to exhibit the same fairly general ideal stride, they are not similar enough to exhibit the same highly specific ideal stride. This is because every person, including a world-class ath-lete, runs in a unique way that cannot be fully duplicated by anybody else.

No Two People Are Alike

When we say "No two people are alike," we are in fact acknowledging a fundamental truth, namely that all of us exhibit differences in perception, sensorimotor patterns (movement), and thus behavior that distinguish each human from every other human on the planet. Obviously, this doesn't mean people are completely unalike. We share general characteristics that we don't with other species, such as chimpanzees, elephants, and slime molds.[8] We even share general patterns of movement and behavior with other individuals and groups of individuals. Beyond the general aspects of our being, however, we are different. And this raises the questions: What exactly are the differences? Do they really matter when it comes to something like running?

To begin with, we normally exhibit at least a few basic anatomical differences when compared to those belonging to not only the opposite sex but other races and ethnic groups. For example: a woman normally possesses a wider pelvic girdle than a man of equal height; For equal height and weight, Africans usually have proportionally longer legs and thus a higher center of mass than Europeans, who, in turn, possess longer legs and thus a higher center of mass than Asians. Gravity ensures that any difference in either pelvic width or center of mass should result in observable differences in at least some basic movement patterns. The pelvic issue, for example, is one reason why we can normally see differences between how a woman walks, runs, and throws a ball as compared to a man.[9] Likewise, when comparing people of equal weight and height, those with a lower center of mass will tend to exhibit less spinal curvature, which in turn may affect the way they perform certain tasks, or at least how they appear when they perform

---

[8] Obviously, at the level of molecular cell biology, we do share some basic attributes with all other forms of life. Many of these attributes are in fact what separate the "quick" from the "dead." Carl Sagan sums up such a perspective nicely: "All organisms on Earth use a kind of molecule called a nucleic acid to encode the hereditary information and to reproduce it in the next generation. All organisms on Earth use the identical code book for translating nucleic acid language into protein language. And while there are clearly some differences between, say, me and a slime mold, fundamentally we are tremendously loosely related. The lesson is, don't judge a book by its cover. At the molecular level, we are all virtually identical." Carl Sagan, *The Varieties of Scientific Experience: A Personal View of the Search for God* (New York: Penguin, 2006), 67.

[9] Differences between the sexes within the structures of the thorax, shoulder girdle, and elbow also play a role in altering gait, stride, and ball-throwing.

them.[10] Whether or not differences in center of mass and thus spinal curvature should play a role in diversifying our notion of ideal posture, gait, or running form has, to my knowledge, yet to be thoroughly examined.

Even taking into account anatomical differences, culture normally plays a far more significant role in affecting our movement styles. The diverse array of movement styles and behavior we see around the world is due in large part to the extraordinary diversity in culture and subculture that exists on our planet. This diversity, which could be attributed to the complex issue of human learning within the context of changing environmental and social conditions, combined with individual-level differences, means that when examined in detail, no two humans move in exactly the same fashion. From the Great Rift Valley to Tierra del Fuego to Easter Island, humanity's millennia-old colonization of every major landmass on the planet could not have occurred without our prodigious learning capacity and thus ability to adapt our culture, way of life, and movement to suit new surroundings. Our ability to learn, in other words, empowers the cultural and social adaptations required to survive in a changing environment; each cultural and social change, in turn, affects what the average person within a particular culture ends up learning. In a circular fashion, learning and culture influence and to some degree circumscribe each other.

Finally, as an integral subset of cultural influence, we cannot ignore the role of child care, which is no longer exclusive to parents, grandparents, and other blood relations but increasingly delegated to wage laborers in the form of day-care employees (or nannies, for children of the wealthy). This shift means the general environment within which each child develops depends not only on the parenting style within the context of the home

---

[10] I am reminded of how different my acture appears from that of my friend Ali when we both configure ourselves into the same basic martial arts stances. Differences in the height of the center of mass mean that the acture for someone of African or African American descent such as Ali should not look exactly the same as the acture for someone of Asian descent such as me. These differences affect not only curvature of the spine but muscle length and girth—one reason Asian boxers often appear to have both larger calf and smaller chest muscles when compared to their European or African counterparts.

environment, but increasingly, on the institutional caretaking style within the context of the ubiquitous day-care center. For just as each style of care-taking influences the child's sensorimotor development in different ways, encouraging or making room for particular explorations while discouraging or removing the possibility for others, each type of physical environment likewise provides unique affordances for a child's exploring and learning. In combination, caretaking style and physical conditions can nurture the child in any general direction of learning and thus any general direction of movement, thought, and behavior.

The Pitfalls of (Over) Correction and Imitation

Given the variables mentioned above that contribute to making each human highly unique, we should naturally expect some problems to stand in our way if our ideal image becomes too specific. For even though experts might direct me toward imitating the stride of any given top-flight runner, the possible benefits accrued in doing so should be limited to how well the given image suits my particular body and mind. The less suitable the match, the less benefit there will be in imitating her stride, and the greater likeli-hood that doing so will have some negative effects—as is the case anytime we try to fit a proverbial square peg into a round hole.[11]

Furthermore, there is the basic question of how accurately and precisely I am actually able to imitate someone else's movement patterns—many to most of which may turn out to be quite novel and therefore foreign to my own nervous system. As I discussed in chapter 8, "Imitation," the more

---

[11] Moshe Feldenkrais puts this concept into a modern social context in the follow-ing statement: "The general tendency toward social improvement in our day has led directly to a disregard, rising to neglect, for the human material of which society is built. The fault lies not in the goal itself but in the fact that individuals, rightly or wrongly, tend to identify their self-images with their value to society. Like a man trying to force a square peg into peculiarities by alienating himself from his inherent needs. He strains to fit himself into the round hole that he now actively desires to fill, for if he fails in this, his value will be so diminished in his own eyes as to discour-age further initiative." Moshe Feldenkrais, *Awareness through Movement* (New York: Harper-Collins, 1990), 18.

sensorimotor awareness, coordination, and thus refined and precise control that goes into performing any given movement pattern, the more sensorimotor awareness, coordination, and thus refined and precise control I will have to have acquired beforehand in order to replicate the pattern with any modicum of accuracy and precision. And this means the greater the difference in sensorimotor awareness between me and the person embodying the ideal image, the less accurate I will be in imitating her or his movements. Thus, if an expert attempts to "fix" my stride by means of simple correction, and in the hope that I will suddenly run more like a world-class runner, unless I already possess a similar level of sensorimotor awareness as that world-class runner, I will end up far off the mark, and consequently experience little to no immediate improvement. If I continue running in this manner, it will be anybody's guess as to how things will end. For the less accurate I am in matching the ideal, the less likely I am to realize predicted gains, and the more likely I am to injure myself over the long run.

Early Childhood

It should go without saying that I cannot realistically expect a few minutes, or even days, of correction to make up for the years of learning that it took for a world-class runner to learn the fundaments of world-class running. For as with all other humans, world-class runners learned the most important aspects of efficient running during the early years of life. In fact, much of their learning occurred on the floor, and in the case of Olympic medalists from places like Bekoji, Ethiopia, Iten, Kenya, and Marobela, Botswana, it occurred on natural terrain, and without impediments to free bodily movement such as stiff or supported shoes, restrictive clothing, and modern restraining devices (strollers, high chairs, Baby Einstein Musical Motion Activity Jumpers, and the like.)[12]

---

[12] If distraction can be considered a form of restraint, electronic devices with screens such as smart phones and tablets also fall into this category.

Finally, it is important to note that in the best of all worlds, infant and toddler sensorimotor learning generally unfolds in an organic, and therefore self-directed, incremental and unselfconscious way. This means that infant-toddler sensorimotor skills develop most efficiently in the absence of outside correction and rigid adherence to ideal images (unless, of course, anxious parents interfere by attempting to artificially speed up the learning process). Such learning is only possible when the individual is not only given the freedom to explore and discover at her own pace but also according to her own inclinations. Obviously, such learning precludes any kind of rigid fixation on a particular ideal.

Only under such conditions does the child have the specific opportunity to more fully explore movement, sense and feel differences within her body, and otherwise collect, differentiate, organize, and reorganize sensorimotor feedback into the neuromuscular patterns we call efficient, graceful, and powerful movement. This sort of "critical sensing," which could be thought of as a precursor to critical thinking, only occurs when the individual has the opportunity to more fully collect, compare, differentiate, organize, reorganize, and otherwise process novel information into the neurological patterns we call knowledge.

An Example from Martial Arts

The issue of accuracy and precision in replicating sensorimotor patterns cuts to a deeper issue that is always lurking beneath the surface when we try to model ourselves on any particular ideal image. While the ideal serves to demonstrate either a more general or more specific image of what we are supposed to look like when we run, it does not, in and of itself, give us many clues as to how we might get there. Fixation on the ideal then tends to lead us to overlook the heart of the matter: If we want to run more efficiently, we must *learn* to run more efficiently; and if we want to learn to run more efficiently, we must know how to learn.

From a neurological perspective, correcting my stride in the hope that it will look like that of a world-class runner generally does not bridge the sensorimotor learning gap that stands between me and actually having the stride of a world-class runner. It does not, in other words, make up for the deficiency in learned sensorimotor awareness that stands between having my stride and having what could be called "world-class stride." While correcting my form or asking me to imitate the current ideal may provide some superficial benefits—especially if the corrections do not overwhelm my nervous system by introducing too much novelty—neither addresses the more fundamental problem of deep learning, something that requires not only a way to directly test the functionality of the correction, but the time, attention, thought, imagination, exploratory impulse, and patience that are all part of the testing.

Perhaps the field of martial arts will help to illustrate the issue more clearly. Good martial arts teachers will devote a good amount of time to guiding beginning students to more stable and otherwise advantageous alignments and positions (advantageous positions, that is, relative to one or more opponents' positions). Such guidance often means examining and correcting the alignment of the entire body when it is frozen in one single moment and under highly specific conditions before moving on to the next moment and set of conditions. Such guidance means, in other words, breaking complex movement sequences into smaller, more digestible parts. Doing so gives the student an opportunity to sense not only how adjustments in any one part can have an effect on all other parts, but how the student must continuously make such adjustments, moment to moment, if her body is to work as a unified system. Moreover, corrections are generally given within the context of improving the functionality of a given martial application. This means that they are given with the context of some kind of sensorimotor feedback by which the student will sense within her body (and in some cases, see with her eyes) whether or not the application is working, and if so, to what degree. This type of correction consequently tests functionality rather than assuming it.

Even without a great deal of instruction, the necessity of making such adjustments becomes more obvious when attempting to throw an opponent (especially if she is simultaneously trying to avoid being thrown), lock an opponent's joint, perform a judo roll or break-fall, escape a joint-lock, strike with some modicum of power, maintain one's balance after evading a blow, maintain one's balance after striking or kicking, maintain one's balance and quickly recover after missing a target, maintain one's balance after getting hit, or practice a choreographed movement sequence (as in a form) in super slow motion while maintaining balance and reversibility. In all of these cases Newtonian physics—the effects of force, acceleration, and gravity on one's body—make it somewhat obvious when a student is losing balance, stability, power, reversibility, and control. It can also help to grossly indicate to the student when she is carrying her spine in a weak alignment, holding parts of herself too flaccidly, or bracing herself too rigidly. Very generally speaking, force, acceleration, gravity, and the student's ability to sense the effects of all three, give her the opportunity to make adjustments, to correct herself, and to learn.[13]

Obviously, none of the above is to say that I will know exactly what adjustments to make or how to make them. Testing functionality, in other words, does not automatically lead to discovery, self-correction, and learning. For me to know what adjustments to make and how to make them requires time, patience, and a willingness to explore and make mistakes. (And in the case of martial arts, it helps if you have training partners who aren't overly committed to inflicting pain on others.) Nonetheless, what testing the functionality of any movement or movement sequence does provide is some modicum of sensory feedback, which is the minimum requirement for discovery, self-correction, and thus learning to take place.

---

[13] Of course, it helps tremendously in the course of learning to have cooperative training partners. Robert W. Smith describes the great potential for learning inherent in the martial art of judo when he writes: "Jigoro Kano envisaged judo as an educative process for the masses of all countries.... He developed this into a system of physical and ethical education. His strategy embraced two ideas: (1) maximum efficiency with minimum effort, and (2) mutual welfare. We have forgotten that the first maxim covered life as well as sport judo and few of us seem to have ever learned the meaning of the second (which means simply love). The *nage* sequence *kuzushi-tsukuri-kake* and other technical prizes developed from sport judo are only tactics that are minor considerations compared with Kano's strategy. Van de Velde, the Dutch gynecologist, said a mouthful when he said that the preliminaries to love are as important as the main event. For without them you can't get from here to there." Robert W. Smith, *Martial Musings: A Portrayal of the Martial Arts in the 20th Century* (Erie, PA: Via Media, 1999), 205.

Whether in martial arts, sports, dance, or other movement domains, corrections are only useful to the degree that a student can sense and feel the consequent changes in her own body—noticing in particular how making an adjustment in one part of her body can result in an adjustment in all other parts of her body, and how this in turn can alter the fundamental way in which she uses herself. Corrections are useful, in other words, to the degree that a student improves her relationship with gravity.

No amount of correction and guidance will by itself bring a student into perfect alignment and positioning. The subtleties of human movement prohibit this from ever occurring, else with the proper corrections, we could all gain mastery of any sport, form of dance, or martial arts with only weeks or even days of expert instruction. While teachers can create opportunities for learning, they cannot gift a student with a more intricate, subtle, and sophisticated awareness of her movement and thereby magically make what could amount to hundreds or even thousands of hours of learning happen in an instant. The student must discover all of this with her own senses, through the same trials and errors by which all masters become masters and by which all world-class runners have acquired the fundaments of efficient running.

In martial arts, the transformation from beginner into intermediate, intermediate into advanced, and so on therefore involves not only precise correction and careful guidance from experienced and knowledgeable teachers who break down movements into smaller, more digestible parts, but the requisite and innumerable trials that enable the student to fully integrate the corrections into her nervous system. The process involves developing not only the sensorimotor patterns that increase power, balance, agility, sensitivity, and speed in a multitude of positions, but those that allow the student to respond optimally to openings, feints, attacks, and counterattacks. The process of learning and improvement involves, therefore, both an ideal model (and the corrections that happen to go along with it), and the innumerable trials with attunement to sensory feedback needed not only to make sense of the corrections but ultimately to test whether the ideal is truly ideal.

Fixation on Ideal Images as a Cultural Problem

Given the time, thought, and effort involved in learning, it should be no surprise that many of the fundamentals for stable, powerful, and agile movement remain misunderstood or ignored and that few students consequently ever get beyond the lowest rungs of proficiency.[14] There are, in fact, strict limitations as to how much learning and thus improvement you can experience when relying exclusively on an ideal image and the corrective measures that will supposedly bring you closer to it.

Going beyond the most superficial levels of understanding in any field requires making sense of the material. It requires, therefore, prolonged periods of sensing, comparing, experimenting, exploring, wondering, thinking, and imagining, all of which collectively give you the opportunity to gradually understand and integrate new information. Thus, what we tend to forget in our fixation on ideal image is that coming closer to or even reaching the ideal, or in some cases, developing a new one, should be the end result of a long and often painstaking learning process, by which we gain a deeper understanding of the subject. If we shoot strictly for the image but miss the substance that stands behind it, we risk becoming a pale, desiccated, and otherwise cheap imitation of what could otherwise be vibrant, real, authentic, and human. We risk possessing only the superficial glimmerings of the subject matter at hand, becoming less a carbon copy of the ideal and more a caricature of it (unless, of course, the ideal is itself an unintended caricature). We risk, finally, overlooking the deficits of the accepted ideal and thereby forgo the possibility of discovering a better one (even if it's only better for ourselves and only under special circumstances).

---

[14] Jeff Haller, Feldenkrais Trainer and the founder of Ideal Organization + Profound Strength, has noted how chronic and sometimes serious injuries among professional athletes, dancers, and martial artists can be traced to their missing subtle yet crucial fundamentals for stable and powerful movement.

Running as a Skill

In contrast to martial arts, the act of running appears to be difficult to break down and "freeze" into digestible frames of movement. Considering that in the act of running both feet are off the ground much of the time, how is it possible for me to freeze my motion in mid-stride? On the face of it, running is a highly complex problem that cannot easily be broken down. On the face of it, we should stick strictly to imitating some ideal image.

Here it is important to reiterate that the fundamental sensorimotor patterns that make a runner world-class were actually learned in childhood, and under particular conditions that afforded opportunities for such learning. World-class runners acquired much of the biomechanical efficiency necessary to make them world-class, in other words, during the process of learning and refining the fundamental sensorimotor patterns necessary for their surviving and gaining independence. The entire process of infant, toddler, and early childhood sensorimotor development, then, contains the building blocks for running. From the earliest explorations by which an infant learns to lift her head to later ones by which she learns to roll over, crawl, and eventually stand, each step in the process is a building block to her eventual striding effortlessly across the finish line. Through engaging all of her senses to explore movement, and given innumerable trials and errors in the process, the infant-toddler-young child creates the sensorimotor, and thus biomechanical, foundation for becoming a world-class runner. Looked at this way, we can see that the problem of breaking down complexity associated with the act of running has already been systematically broken down, examined, and understood to one degree or another by that group of prototypical biomechanics researchers otherwise known as children.

Conventional Analysis of Stride

In the last few years I have seen more than a few YouTube videos where running experts analyze the stride of world-class runners in order to demonstrate what the correct way of running looks like. Some go as far as to compare the movements of the top-place holders in races involving some of the world's best runners in order to expose the supposed flaws exhibited by those who came in second, third, or slightly farther back in the field. The implication here is that if number two and three had only run more correctly (more like the winner of the race), they would have performed better and possibly beaten number one. Taken to its logical conclusion, we should be looking for faults in the stride of anyone who is neither the winner of a particular important race, nor the current world record holder. We should assume, in other words, that everyone but the winner is flawed, and that a highly specific ideal image—namely the one exhibited by the winner—is suitable for everyone. Yet, even if this were true, it still does not address how the winner acquired her ideal stride. Unless we address the deep learning by which the acquisition took place, such infinitesimal dissection of what is "correct" versus what is "incorrect" will leave us with no compass by which to direct us toward our desired destination.

These days, it seems that everybody is fair game when it comes to comparisons with the fashionable ideal such that even the reigning world champion and world record holder could use a bit of advice. Before Usain Bolt's retirement from track and field, former 200-meter and 400-meter world record holder Michael Johnson, for example, announced on separate television broadcasts that Bolt could lower his world record times for the 100- and 200-meter dash if he would only "clean up" his technique, and run more perfectly—more, incidentally, like Johnson.[15] His evidence is based on Bolt's supposed biomechanical flaws, all of which Johnson points out while reviewing film footage of Bolt's record-setting performances.

---

[15] In one broadcast, Johnson insinuates that he himself exhibits the ideal stride. Earlier in the same broadcast he flatly states, "We don't think of ourselves as machines, but in many ways that is how we perform, how we move." Stephen Lyle and Leon Mann, directors, *Usain Bolt: The Fastest Man Who Has Ever Lived*, BBC 2 television, May 15, 2010. In an article for Slate titled "Making the Perfect Sprinter More Perfect: How Usain Bolt Could Have Run Even Faster" (August 5, 2017), Adam Willis states, "Former 200- and 400-meter world record holder Michael Johnson has said Bolt could run 9.4 in the 100 and break 19 in the 200 if he cleaned up his form. 'Technically he is not the best. Technically he is a bit all over the place,' Johnson said in 2014. Johnson elaborated to the BBC at the 2015 world championships, critiquing Bolt's upper-body movement: 'He doesn't have lateral stability, so you will see a lot of rocking back and forth.' He also criticized Bolt's starts, saying that the sprinter is 'clunky' and 'all over the place' when he comes out of the blocks."

Yet, is it really true, as the old bromide goes, that there is always room for betterment and (self-) improvement? If so, does everyone necessarily get better when they attempt to copy the latest fashionable ideal? Should Usain Bolt, for example, consider going to Michael Johnson's running clinic? Should second- and third-place finishers in an Olympic final "correct" their stride so that they run more like the first-place finishers? And should we therefore ignore the myriad other factors that can influence race results, such as illness, injury, illicit doping, strategic mistakes, overtraining, peaking at the wrong time, mental fatigue, experiencing an off day, or the effects of aging, to name just a few? Should we, who are not even close to approaching the ability of a world-class runner, heed the implication that our grievous defects would be at least partially solved by copying, or at least attempting to copy, the "proper" form?

I, for one, am not convinced that such infinitesimal dissection is always necessary or even useful. While a relatively *general* ideal image may be essential for learning and improvement, being either too specific in defining the image or too rigid in pursuing conformity to it can direct us away from the kind of exploration that can lead to discovery. Besides that, human movement is extraordinarily complex—too complex in fact, for there to be only one highly specific model for proper stride. Furthermore, suggesting that through biomechanical analysis we can know exactly where someone's flaws are, and exactly how, therefore, they could be fixed, is putting undue faith in the diagnostic precision of biomechanics. Moreover, with or without biomechanics, we are still left with the issue of how one acquires a more efficient stride even if we know (generally) what an ideal one might look like. Does, for example, the acquisition occur by correcting? Imitating? Some combination of the two? If "yes" to any of the above, where does learning fit into the picture?

Humans, Machines, and Biomechanics

It is important to note that the field of biomechanics arose from mechanics, which is in large part the study of what happens when force is applied to inanimate objects. As the industrial age brought machines into the picture, scientists began applying mechanics to machine movement. Only more recently have the principles of mechanics been brought to humans.

While applying mechanics to machine movement has to some degree worked out relatively smoothly, the step from machines to humans has proven to be problematic for a few reasons. Because even the most sophisticated machines exhibit far fewer degrees of freedom than living, breathing creatures such as human beings, their movement is far less complex and far easier to analyze and generalize. Consequently, unlike human movement, machine movement generally follows a repetitive, narrow, fixed, and in the case of robotics, preprogrammed protocol. With some exceptions, any variation in the movement of any part of a machine is thus generally left to a human controller. More complex machines may be able to vary their tasks independently, but the degrees of freedom of which they are in control are still minimal compared to the number contained in the human organism.

All of this means that control systems used for machines are far less complex than that of the human control system otherwise known as the human brain and nervous system. For unlike machine movement, which with few exceptions tends to be highly restricted, repetitive, and unvarying, human movement varies greatly. The many degrees of freedom available in the human body and the consequent number of possible variations with which any movement can be performed means that each person carries her own unique way of moving that not only *is not*, but *cannot* be shared to a high level of specificity with any other person on the planet. Herein lies the problem.

In order to bring the field of mechanics into the living world and thereby make it *bio*mechanics, engineers must radically simplify human movement by dramatically reducing degrees of freedom, effectively reducing the representation of the human body to a collection of points, lines, and levers. The result thus far is to produce a fairly vague and general understanding of ideal movement rather than a precise and specific one. Moreover, simplifying and otherwise reducing human movement reduces some of the human aspects of movement and makes it more machinelike.

Unfortunately, most attempts to make runners more biomechanically efficient amount to correcting their form in the hope that they will run more like somebody with an ideal stride. That is, "input correction A, and you get the desired output B." Yet, the complexity of the human body—or more aptly put, *bodymind*—including not only its myriad degrees of freedom but also the extraordinarily complex nervous system controlling those degrees—means that improving movement is a highly complex affair that cannot be solved by providing a list of standard corrections. Unlike machines, we do not function by simple "input-output" formulas. For as I mentioned earlier, the greater the difference between my stride and the ideal, the more piecemeal exploration and learning I must undertake in order to make up for that difference. The greater the difference between my stride and the ideal, the more any correction, no matter how apparently simple, will be impossible to integrate into the movement of my entire body without a good deal of exploration. And as I mentioned earlier, this means it is impossible to instantaneously incorporate a foreign sensorimotor pattern without first having learned and incorporated the sensorimotor building blocks that make the pattern possible.

The normal recourse in such cases of sensorimotor disparity is to attempt to imitate the "proper" movement or positioning of one or more parts of the body—for example, the knees, arms, head, or chest—without sensing and feeling in one's own body and thereby fully understanding that it is the complex *relationship* between the moment-to-moment movement (or positioning) of each part of the body with the moment-to-moment movement (or positioning) of the entire rest of the body that is crucial. Efficient positioning and efficient movement are, in a sense, the result of an ultimately cooperative relationship between each part of the body and the entire whole, as that whole moves within the context of an ever-changing environment. It follows that efficient movement means that no part of the body works in isolation. Each part acts instead as one link in a biomechanically sound pattern involving the entire body, from head to literal toe.

Increasing Awareness

Given what I've stated above, I think it is important to clarify the difference between corrections that improve sensorimotor awareness and those that don't. A useful correction will give me greater insight into, and awareness of, what my habits are and how I might go about finding better ones. If corrections are provided incrementally in small enough doses that they don't overwhelm my nervous system, and if I am given the time and opportunity for my entire body to sense, feel, and respond to the novel stimuli, I have the chance of gaining more awareness. If, on the other hand, I do not have the time and opportunity to integrate the novel stimuli, the correction will probably not lead to greater self-awareness, which means that it will probably not lead to any improvement. And corrections that do not increase my awareness will tend to make me less independent and more reliant on external referents to tell me what to do. For if I cannot sense how a given correction can be integrated into the movement of my entire body, I cannot truly know whether or not the correction improves my movement. And if I cannot know, then I must rely on somebody else who supposedly does.

Obviously, some sort of ideal image and form of correction are both important, and some would say, vital for learning. The type of education that places too much of a premium on conforming to an ideal image, however, will tend to do so at the expense of exploring, wondering, and increasing awareness, thereby sacrificing deeper learning in the process. At the extremes, attempting to fit people into a preset mold, as fixation on a particular ideal image tends to do, can work to the detriment of awareness, a deeper understanding, and even a deeper sense of self.

Finally, because fixating on an ideal image can at times prevent an individual from discovering her own way—one which might be better suited to her own idiosyncrasies and consequently more effective at producing the desired results—doing so can, in certain cases, also detract from performance. As my friend and esteemed colleague John Cedric Tarr so aptly observed, to have "improved" Usain Bolt's stride, supposedly making him more biomechanically efficient by conforming to Michael Johnson's ideal, might have meant destroying much of what made him *him*. I would add that having done so would have also eliminated precisely what made him a nine-time Olympic champion.

We Are Born to Learn (and to Run)

Through tireless play, endless exploration, and innumerable trials, the suckling newborn gradually develops into the crawling baby, who in turn grows into the teetering toddler, and eventually the scampering child. With each step in the process, the infant-toddler-child acquires the sensorimotor patterns that form the foundation for the next phase of development. With each step, she continues to pour the foundation for increasingly complex motor skills, including the skill known as running.

Given the disparity in efficiency between the stride of an average runner and that of a world-class runner, it is important for those of us who want to improve to reexamine the foundation of sensorimotor skills upon which our own stride has been built. With this in mind, we may want to return to some of the basic explorations from childhood in order to recapture the patterns that have been lost over the years, or more likely, were never acquired in the first place. We may want, in short, to regain our senses by exploring movement in any number of configurations while using any number of constraints our imagination can conjure up.

Sensing, feeling, experimenting, or in a word, exploring, are precisely all we have as humans if we want to make deep improvements in anything. The type of deep learning by which all world-class runners first gained both economy of motion and power in their stride is not only how all of us learned to put one foot in front of the other, but how all of us could learn to do so far more efficiently, powerfully, painlessly, effortlessly, even joyfully. Counterintuitively, attempting to match a particular ideal without more fully understanding how the ideal came into being in the first place will, more often than not, lead us away from the deep learning that would otherwise bring us closer to the ideal. And if attachment to an ideal becomes too strong, it may prevent us from sensing, feeling, and thinking for ourselves, and consequently discovering the possible *less-than-ideal* aspects of the ideal.

When so many are offering quick and easy ways to improve your running, when following a handful of expert tips will supposedly increase your speed while at the same time make your stride feel effortless, when the science of biomechanics can, according to some, tell you exactly how to run like a champion, spending time to explore movement may seem rather ordinary, boring, and even useless. In a culture where promises of fast and miraculous results have become all too common, the idea of slowing down in order to (re)learn how to run will feel as uninteresting to most as the notion of deep learning will seem unpalatable, if not entirely alien. Yet, rarely, if ever, do profound, meaningful, and lasting changes occur overnight, or in the time it takes to complete an online master class taught by a famous instructor, or even in the time it takes to complete a weeklong retreat (even if it's taught by the same instructor and held in an exclusive tropical resort offering daily poolside massages). Learning itself is incremental: a series of small steps that over a long period of time can lead to deep knowledge and profound understanding.

A

The Feldenkrais Method

Free choice is meaningless when we are compelled to adopt the one and only way we know.

—MOSHE FELDENKRAIS

The Feldenkrais Method was born out of a childlike curiosity that all of us possess, even if, for most of us, it lies buried beneath several layers of conformity. Its founder, Moshe Feldenkrais, exemplified the same fiercely independent way of thinking that we see in all great scientists, musicians, artists, writers, dancers, and athletes—indeed, anyone who values exploration, uncertainty, and playfulness. It is also the same sort of mindset that we see in infants, toddlers, and young children and that we ourselves embody in our more spontaneous, less defensive, and perhaps more vulnerable moments.

Born in Ukraine in 1904, Feldenkrais traveled on foot and alone to what is now Israel at the age of fourteen. Several years later he attended the Sorbonne in Paris and began working toward his doctorate in mechanical engineering under Frédéric Joliot-Curie, the 1935 Nobel Prize winner in chemistry. While at the Sorbonne, Feldenkrais met Jigoro Kano, the distinguished Japanese physicist and founder of judo.

At its highest levels, judo is dominated by those who are least reliant on brute force and therefore, most persistent in listening, searching, and adapting—those, in other words, who put learning above winning. In this regard, judo, which means "the gentle way" (and whose greatest masters could therefore be considered quintessential gentlewomen and gentlemen), can be considered the art of cultivating sense-ability.[1] In *Martial Musings,* Robert W. Smith writes:

> Kano envisaged judo as an educative process for the masses of all countries.... He developed this into a system of physical and ethical education. His strategy embraced two ideas: (1) maximum efficiency with minimum effort, and (2) mutual welfare. We have forgotten that the first maxim covered life as well as sport judo and few of us seem to have ever learned the meaning of the second (which means simply love).

After meeting Kano, Feldenkrais, a high-level martial artist himself, immersed himself in the study of judo, and quickly rose in the European ranks. Seeing judo's vast potential to further growth and human development, he later wrote several important books on the art. Human development through exploring movement, or what he called "awareness through movement," was to become a major theme in Feldenkrais's later work.

---

[1] Indeed, any discipline can become a medium for cultivating sense-ability. Renowned Belgian soccer coach Michel Bruyninckx, for example, uses soccer for just this purpose. He expresses his sensible approach as follows: "I create players that can play to win at the right moment, but firstly you have to explain that learning is more important than winning games." John Sinnott, "Cracking Coaching's Final Frontier," BBC Sport, March 22, 2011.

B

The Lessons

What's in the Lessons?

Each of the twenty-seven lessons works with one or more of the following four themes: (1) waking up your feet and legs; (2) connecting your hands to your pelvis, legs, and feet through the flexing, extending, rotating, and side-bending of your spine (i.e., coordinating the movement of your extremities with that of your spine as it traverses one, two, or all three planes of motion); (3) shedding light on the hidden yet crucial aspect of what's happening behind you as you run; (4) stabilizing and elongating your spine. I chose these themes for the following reasons:

Most runners I know have weak feet and legs. The major reason for this is that like me, they grew up in a culture where people normally sit in chairs instead of on the floor, wear heavily supported shoes, and walk on flat pavement. The entire "Throwing the Ball" series (Lessons 1–9) along with Lessons 18, 19, and 22–25 are designed in part to help to wake up your feet and legs.

Your hands, arms, and shoulders are obviously important for running, but to generate more power in your stride, you must know what to do with them. Lessons 2, 3, 9, 11, 12, 17, and 27, along with the entire "Metatarsals to Metacarpals" series (Lessons 21–26) will help you understand how to generate far greater power by coordinating the movement of your hands, arms, and shoulders with the varied and intricate articulations in your spine, pelvis, legs, and feet.

Half of your stride occurs behind your rear end and behind your back. When we say to someone, "lift your knees higher," we are showing our attentive bias toward everything that occurs in front of us and within our field of vision. The result of such a bias is to tend to neglect everything outside our field of vision, even though what is outside of it may play a crucial role in determining what is happening inside of it. Five lessons in particular (10, 11, 13, 22, and 23) will help you discover how much more power you gain once you begin to connect your back to your front (as well as your bottom to your top, and your left to your right).

When you are running, you want your spine to be pliable but not floppy; elongated and stable, but not stiff. Watch Olympic runners and you can get a sense of both stability and elongation. Notice how tall they look as they stride down the track. Lessons 9, 10, 12, 14, 15, 20, and 26 are among the lessons that will help you to discover what it means to have an elongated and stable spine.

Things to Keep in Mind ...

If you hit a million balls against a backboard, and are inattentive or bored, your arm may grow stronger, but your awareness won't, and little will be learned; in fact, you may not even recognize that you're bored and playing a game you don't enjoy.

—W. TIMOTHY GALLWEY, *INNER TENNIS*

Go Slowly

Unless otherwise instructed, go slowly so that you can be more attentive and feel what is happening in your body. Change your pace from time to time, noticing how going slower or faster affects your ability to sense the fine details in your movement.

No Pain = More Gain (at Least Most of the Time)

Stop if anything hurts or if you feel like you are straining. Learning occurs much faster when you are not distracted by discomfort and can give your full attention to what you are doing. Doing anything without your full attention, on the other hand, generally stifles progress. Straining or pushing to the point of discomfort in any capacity—whether physical or emotional—tends to block your mind from getting new information. Some lessons, such as ones from the "Throwing the Ball" series, will be challenging at first, leading certain muscles to tire quickly. I recommend you not push yourself during these lessons because your precision will suffer as a result. As I have suggested many times in this book, you get more out of things when you stop trying to get more out of them.

No Pain, No Gain (under Particular Circumstances)

Under certain conditions, it can be beneficial to push yourself. Lessons 18 and 19, for example, are intended to present a physical challenge. Unlike with the other lessons, I consequently encourage you to incrementally test your conditioning during the final steps of these lessons.

Notice if You Feel Bored or Frustrated

Stop if at any point you feel frustrated or even bored. You are better off resting or even doing something else if you feel either of these. Discomfort, strain, frustration, and boredom are the greatest saboteurs of learning.

Rest Frequently

Don't wait until you are tired before stopping. It isn't the number of repetitions you perform that matters, but whether you are becoming more precise in your ability to sense your own movement. Improving precision depends crucially on resting periodically.

Bookmark for Later

Some lessons, like Lessons 7, 12, 22, and 23, may present a serious challenge to your flexibility. If you feel intense stretching, particularly in your feet, knees, hips, neck, or back, or if you feel any strain, particularly in your neck, back, or knees, it's a sign that you've gone way too far. Consider skipping parts of or even entire lessons if they feel risky. Save them for later, or break them into smaller pieces, working perhaps with just one or two steps of a lesson at a time, rather than trying to tackle the whole lesson at once.[1]

Savor New Sensations ... Do a Body Scan

Scan yourself before and after each lesson (and if you want, during rest periods). This way you will start to notice subtle changes in your body. These changes are an indication of neurological change also known as learning. They are what will guide you to more power, speed, agility, and fluidity. Furthermore, they will enhance your enjoyment.

Be Playful

After you've completed an entire lesson, it isn't necessary to start from the beginning. Feel free to skip around. Whatever step in the lesson you go to, the key is to be attentive, playful, and exploratory.

---

[1] When one series of lessons that I encountered during my Feldenkrais training was simply too difficult for me to finish the first time around, I ended up bookmarking it as something to attempt in the future. When well over a decade later I decided to give it another try, it took several weeks of daily work to get through all of the lessons in their entirety. As I continued to go farther, working with specific parts of the lessons for a series of months, I began to realize that the explorations I was engaging in were not only rehabilitating my injured right knee but realigning my spine at the same time. Naturally, my gait and stride began to feel lighter and more powerful as a result. Had I rushed through the series this second time around, gone for the deep stretch at the outset, and otherwise performed the lessons rather than exploring them gently and at my own pace, I'm certain that I would have further aggravated my knee while forgoing the potential benefits of the lessons.

Close Your Eyes (When Appropriate)

For lessons where you are lying down or sitting, I recommend keeping your eyes closed unless otherwise directed. Closing your eyes tends to diffuse your focus and thereby free up your neck muscles. It also helps you to direct your attention to what you are sensing and feeling. For standing lessons, I recommend keeping your eyes open, unless otherwise instructed.

Work with Friends

Humans are social animals. Not only do we tend to learn more effectively when meeting periodically in groups, but we fulfill our primal need for social bonding. Given this, I encourage you to gather with others on a regular basis in order to explore lessons together.

Lessons 1–9
"Throwing the Ball" Series

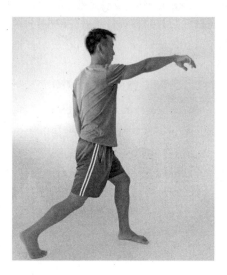

The "Throwing the Ball" series will help you develop particular movement patterns used by Bagua adepts and many professional athletes. The starting positions may seem unusual and challenging at first, since these lessons are meant to arouse areas in your body that have been dormant for years and possibly decades. As your body awakens and your sense-abilities improve, what was at first challenging will quickly become easier. The reason is that rather than simply working harder at habitual movements, you will be working smarter by exploring novel movements.

Each of the lessons is meant to build power through coordination, which is why it is possible to feel significant improvements in both posture and propulsive force in a relatively short period of time. Devoting 20–30 minutes every day to "Throwing the Ball" lessons can lead to noticeable changes by the end of the week. By the seventh day, what once seemed very difficult will likely seem manageable and probably much easier. Of course, consistency in exploring lessons over a longer period of time—say a month to six months—will lead to far greater improvements.

Finally, for all the lessons that involve standing, I recommend using a full-length mirror from time to time to check both your beginning and ending positions. The mirror can help you become aware of what you wouldn't otherwise notice, such as when you start leaning forward or bending sideways. Videotaping can be even more powerful because it allows you to see even more of what you wouldn't otherwise notice about your own movement.

Lesson 1
Posing Questions

Starting Position: Take off your shoes and stand with your body facing an imaginary target. Have your feet about hip-width apart.

1. Place an imaginary tennis ball in your hand, then step forward and throw the ball. How far forward do you step? Which way is your front foot pointing? Try it several times, altering the amount of force you want to employ.

   A. Which foot do you step with?

   B. Experiment with how far you step and where the foot points.

   C. If you haven't done so already, make sure that you are stepping with the foot opposite your throwing arm. Thus, if you are throwing with your left hand, step forward with your right foot.

   D. Notice that the softer your throw, the smaller the step. The harder and faster the throw, the larger your step will likely be.

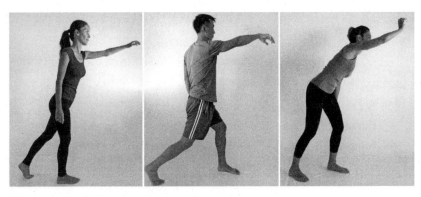

Which position looks more balanced?

2. Now continue to throw a little harder with each throw. Continue until you're throwing with a decent amount of force—as if you wanted to deliver the ball quickly to a target twenty or thirty yards away.

3. Begin to freeze at the very end of your throw and notice how much balance you have. Make sure you don't lift your back foot off the floor.

   A. How long could you stand this way without toppling? How relaxed is your throwing shoulder?

   B. Which way is your front foot pointing? Straight? At an angle to the right or left?

   C. Where is your front knee relative to your front ankle? In front, back, or directly over it?

   D. Note that people encountering this lesson for the first time will often lean forward with their upper body, believing that this will afford them more power. Some will push their front knee forward as they simulate the throw. Either of these strategies will not only reduce power but likely increase the amount of strain on the knee and back.

4. Here we arrive at some basic questions:

   A. What is a more optimal direction for your front foot to be pointing?

   B. How can you perform the action without leaning forward?

   C. How can you perform it without your left knee going forward, yet still gain power?

   D. What would happen if your front knee moved backward (without straightening) as your throwing hand moved forward?

5. It can be illuminating to search for a variety of solutions to even the most basic questions like the ones posed above. In just a few minutes, the searching can reveal a tremendous amount. From a neurophysiological standpoint, the experimentation that often follows this type of searching leads to the development of a host of

new neural connections. Furthermore, the seeking and experimenting can be like deciphering the possible meanings embedded in a good poem, film, or piece of art; each time you return to any given lesson, even if you have already explored it an untold number of times, there is the possibility of discovering something new.

6. Take a break for as long as you want to think about the questions—seconds, minutes, hours, or even days—then try this lesson again.

7. Whenever you are ready, explore the lesson on the other side (throwing with your opposite hand).

Lesson 2
Screwing Foot into Wall[2]

Starting Position: Lie down on your left side with your left foot resting on the floor—the entire sole against the wall. If you need support under your head, fold bath towels neatly and stack them under your left cheek. Make sure that your left foot is far enough forward so that you can see your ankle (your left knee will be bent). Reach down with your fingers and locate the joint that connects your right big toe to the ball of your foot. We'll call this the 1st metatarsal joint. Squeeze it firmly from both the top and the bottom so that you can feel it clearly, and then let go and rest your right hand on top of your left hand (as shown in the image below).

Place your right foot on the wall about one foot behind your body and about two feet off the floor. Lift your heel and the outside edge of your foot so that only the 1st metatarsal joint of your foot is touching the wall. Lift all of your toes so that, except for your big toe, no others are in contact with the wall.

---

[2] This lesson is inspired in part by the work of Ruthy Alon. Ruthy is the founder of Bones for Life and the author of *Mindful Spontaneity: Lessons in the Feldenkrais Method* (Berkeley, CA: North Atlantic Books, 1996). For another take on some of the rotational concepts in this lesson, go to Lesson 17, "Reach and Roll on Your Back," or Lesson 27, "Where Does My Arm Begin? (Reach and Roll on Your Side)."

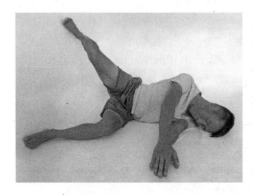
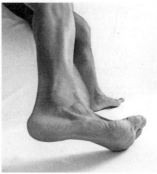

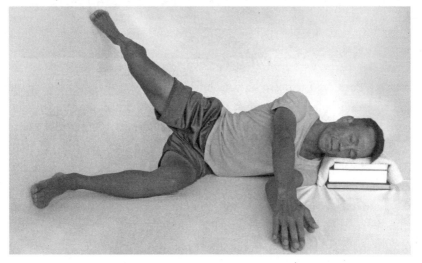

Keep in mind that you can always use firm supports under your head if doing so allows you to be more comfortable.

1. Begin to rotate as if to crush out a cigarette. Notice how your right hip moves as you do this. Go back and forth slowly a few times.

   A. Be very observant of keeping everything but the 1st metatarsal joint off the wall.

   B. Notice when the outside edge of your right foot starts to drop such that the 2nd or 3rd metatarsal joints begin to touch the wall.[3]

---

[3] If your 1st metatarsal joint is sensitive, and pressing from here causes pain, try substituting with the 2nd metatarsal joint or the area between the 1st and the 2nd joint.

2. Now rotate farther forward, and notice what prevents you from going farther. Again, be vigilant that the outside edge of your right foot and everything but your 1st metatarsal and big toe stay away from the wall. Repeat a few times, then pause.

A. Now as you crush out the cigarette, see to it that your right hip rolls forward at the same time.

B. Begin to carefully synchronize the rolling of your right hip with the rotation of your right foot. Repeat a few times, each time noticing when the foot and pelvis are out of sync.

C. Rest on your back.

3. Return to the same configuration, and this time, as you rotate your foot and pelvis, simultaneously turn your head to look to your left—that is, toward the floor.

A. See to it that you move your head more and more in synchrony with the movement of your leg. Go slowly enough to notice when your head begins to move faster than your leg, or when your leg begins to move faster than your head.

B. Repeat this a few times and rest on your back.

4. In resting, notice if you feel like half of your body is sinking more into the floor, or if the floor is tilting to one side. This could be an indication that the muscles on one side of you have given up some of their extraneous tension.

5. Come back to the same configuration, and this time begin to slide your top hand away from you as if trying to reach something on the floor just beyond your fingertips. Start with a very small movement.

A. As you slide forward, notice if your leg moves as well. Notice when other parts of your foot start to make contact with the wall—again, only the big toe and 1st metatarsal joint should be in contact with the wall.

B. Close your eyes and allow your head to roll on the floor as you reach forward. As long as you go slowly, this will help to release the muscles in your neck. As a result, the movement may feel quite soothing. As your body gets more in sync, everything from head to toe will literally move at the same time. Repeat this a few times.

C. Now try leading once with the rotation of your right foot to see if your leg, hand, and arm follow. Keep your eyes closed. Is your head rolling easily on the floor?

D. Try leading once by gently rolling your head to see if your hand and foot follow.

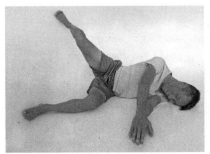 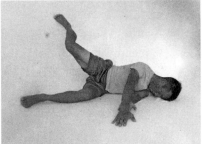

Left: neutral; right: reaching forward.

E. Alternate between leading with your head, hand, and foot, each time checking to see if the other parts of you are moving in synchrony. When you are finished exploring, rest on your back and notice if the two sides of your body feel even more different than before (perhaps one side is sinking even more).

6. Begin to crush the cigarette by rotating your foot in the opposite direction.

A. Make only small movements, and sense the movement in the right side of your pelvis. Notice if your right shoulder is moving.

B. Synchronize the movement such that the right side of your pelvis rolls backward as your foot turns outward (laterally), and it rolls forward as your foot returns to neutral.

C. Start to sense the movement in your chest and in your right shoulder. Is your right hand moving at all? What is your head doing?

D. Continue going back and forth, leading with the rotation of your right foot. Rest when you are ready.

7. Continue rotating your foot outward and back to neutral. This time pay attention to how your head is moving.

A. For every degree your foot rotates, you should sense some response in your head and neck.

B. Go back and forth slowly a few times, every now and then noticing if you are holding your breath.

C. Pause, and begin to lead the movement with your head: as your head turns toward the ceiling, your foot should be rotating outward. Coordinate the movement carefully such that the head and foot move more closely in synchrony.

D. Go back and forth a few times, leading with your head, then resume leading with your foot.

E. Rest.

8. Continue rotating your foot outward and then back to neutral. This time bring your attention to your top hand. Notice if it slides backward as you rotate your foot.

A. Go back and forth once or twice, then pause and begin to lead the movement with your hand: as your hand slides backward, see to it that your foot simultaneously rotates outward. As your hand slides forward, your foot will rotate inward.

B. Alternate between leading with either your hand or your foot.

C. Rest on your back after a couple of iterations.

9. Repeat steps 1 to 8, but this time press into the wall with only your 2nd metatarsal. To make this possible, use masking tape to secure

some small coins to the wall and press the 2nd metatarsal joint of your right foot against them. Lift your heel, and as much as possible, all your toes and all but the 2nd metatarsal joint from the wall. Notice how shifting to your 2nd metatarsal shifts your range of rotation: it reduces internal rotation, but increases external rotation.

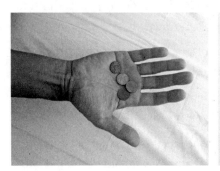 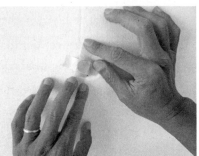

Coins taped to the wall serve as a focal point.

10. When you are finished exploring the relation between your 2nd metatarsal and the movement of your hip, head, and hand, move on to your 3rd, then your 4th, and finally your 5th metatarsal.

    A. Notice how your range of internal and external rotation shifts depending on which metatarsal you are pressing into the wall (and thus, which metatarsals are lifting from the wall). Rotating solely on the 1st metatarsal while lifting all the toes maximizes your range of internal rotation while minimizing your range of external rotation. Conversely, rotating solely on the 5th metatarsal while lifting all the toes minimizes your range of internal rotation while maximizing your range of external rotation.

    B. When you are finished exploring, rest on your back and notice the marked difference between your right and left sides. One leg will probably feel much longer, one foot much larger. Even your two arms and hands will feel quite different from each

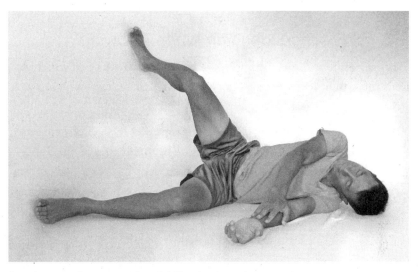

Rotating your foot outward and rolling backward.

other. If you are very attentive, you will notice that the two sides of your face feel different. See if you can describe the differences.

C. The perceived differences will be even more accentuated when you stand up.

11. Stand up and walk around. You will likely notice that your gait is very uneven. One foot likely rolls off the floor with greater clarity and power. One hip will feel more open and free, extending in a way as to generate more propulsive force.

A. If it calls to you, take a walk around your neighborhood and enjoy the changes that have occurred as a result of your explorations.

B. You might even consider running around the block to see how differently your two hips extend, among other differences.

12. Repeat steps 1 to 11 on the other side. (Note that it is not necessary to complete this lesson all at once. Feel free to take time off and resume at another hour or even on another day.)

Lesson 3
Flexing/Extending While Throwing[4]

Starting Position: Throw the imaginary ball once or twice using either arm. Remember to have the opposite foot forward. After a few tries, drop your arms, leaving your feet where they are.

1. Imagine a smoldering cigarette resting under the ball of your back foot. Begin to crush out the cigarette by rotating that foot. Notice the movement of your knee and hip. It's possible other parts of you will also be rotating. Which part(s) of the ball of your foot are you rotating on? Specifically, which metatarsals make contact with the floor? Pause.

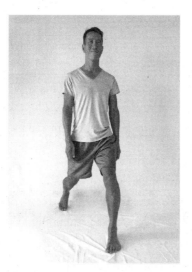
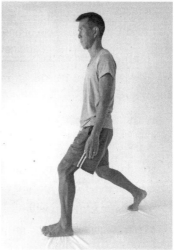

A. Go back and forth taking note of different aspects of your movement, including if and when you begin to lose your balance, and which way your front foot is pointed. Don't be afraid

---

[4] This lesson is closely related to Lesson 5, "Flexing/Extending While Throwing in Sitting," and Lesson 9, "Reaching Up While Throwing."

to adjust the positioning of either or both feet. In fact, consider widening your stance if it is narrow.

B. When you rotate the back foot, does your pelvis also rotate? If not, intentionally start to rotate it. In fact, begin to synchronize the rotation of your pelvis with the rotation of your foot. See to it that neither moves faster than the other.

C. Go slowly so that you can notice when you are getting out of sync.

D. Rest whenever you want.

2. Resume the ball-throwing position, letting your arms rest at your sides. Begin to raise your tailbone such that you feel your lower back arching more. Raise it higher and higher, exaggerating the motion until you feel your back very hyperextended. At the same time, pull your shoulders back so that your chest protrudes forward and upward.

A. When you have reached the comfortable limit to lifting your tailbone, reverse the motion and begin to drop your tailbone. Simultaneously, allow your chest to follow; it will begin to sink downward and backward. If you continue the motion, you will feel your tailbone tucking under you and your trunk moving toward the fetal position.

B. Go back and forth between comfortable extremes of extension and flexion, synchronizing the lifting-dropping of your tailbone with the opening-closing of your chest.

C. Rest.

3. Continue the previous exploration, going back and forth between extreme flexion and extreme extension.

A. Freeze in extreme extension, and in this position, begin to rotate on your back foot again.

B. Go back and forth, sensing what it's like to rotate with your spine and pelvis in this configuration. Notice what is happening in your hip joint and the muscles around it.

C. Rest after a few iterations.

4. Return to the throwing position and gradually bring your trunk into full flexion such that your chest is in and your tailbone is tucked. Begin to turn your back foot.

A. Notice how different the motion is when you are in a highly flexed configuration.

B. Go back and forth noting how different the rotation is as compared to being in an extended position.

C. Rest.

5. In the throwing position, begin to sink your chest in slowly and then begin to protrude it slowly. Synchronize the movement of your chest with that of your tailbone such that neither moves faster than the other. Go back and forth.

A. Go very slowly and begin to note when your lower back is flat—that is, when it feels neither extended nor flexed. In this position the lower back should feel long and your chest will be slightly sunken. You may feel slightly slouched.

B. Once you have found this position, stay there and begin to rotate on your back foot again, noticing how different it feels compared to when you were exploring the motion in the previous configurations.

C. Rest after a few trials.

6. Go back to throwing an imaginary ball and notice how the motion has changed. Are you more stable? Do you feel more power in your throw?

A. Walk a little and notice the propulsion you feel when rolling off your right foot.

B. You will probably also feel more rotation in your trunk and that you are clearly leading with one of your shoulders when you walk.

7. Take some time to enjoy the asymmetry of your gait before repeating steps 1 to 6 on the other side. When you are finished, notice what is different about your posture and gait.

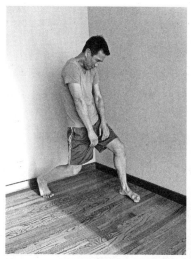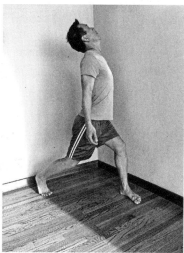

Left: extreme flexion; right: extreme extension.

Lesson 4
Stabilizing Your Front Leg While Lying Down

Starting Position: Lie on your back with your rear end about one foot from the wall—close enough that you can place the sole of your left foot against it while your knee is bent. (Obviously, if you have relatively long legs, lie farther away from the wall, and if you have shorter legs, lie closer.)

Comfortably fold your right leg underneath—let it rest so that your right foot is somewhere between your right buttock and the wall and your knee is turned out to the right. (Place cushions under your right knee if you feel any pulling in your groin muscles.)

1. In this position, bring your left foot as close to the floor as possible while keeping the toes pointing toward the ceiling. The closer you come to the floor, the more your heel will lift.

2. Pretend that the wall is a garage door that slides up and down. Begin to push your left foot into this door as if you wanted to slide it up. (This lesson is better to do without socks so that your foot doesn't slide.) Push with gradually increasing force and then

release just as slowly. Repeat a few times. Notice which muscles in your leg begin to work. Notice if there is a strain in your left knee. How much power do you have in raising the garage door? What effect is there on your left hip? Do you feel movement in your spine?

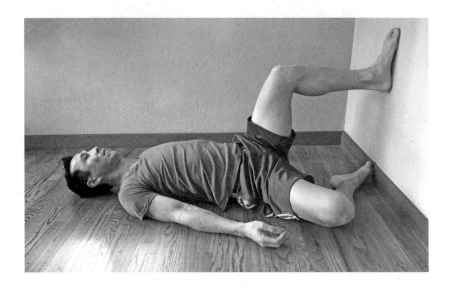

3. Slide your foot three inches higher and repeat. Your heel should be closer to the wall now if it isn't already touching it. Do you get more comfort and power in this position or the previous one with your foot closer to the floor?

4. Slide your foot another three inches higher and repeat. Notice how the higher you place your foot on the wall, the more pressure you exert with your heel, and the more power you get.[5] Notice how your hips and spine are affected differently as you place your foot higher.

---

[5] Because the heel is higher than the midsole in the vast majority of shoes, most peoples' calf muscles are overworked, short, and tight. This lesson will help to lengthen the calf muscles and activate other areas in your legs to help produce more power and balance while stabilizing your knees.

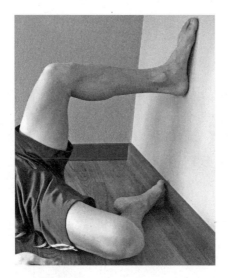

5. Continue placing your foot higher up the ceiling and attempting to slide the imaginary garage door, noticing what's happening in your foot, knee, and hip.

   A. Each height simulates a different way to use your front leg when throwing a ball, or reversing or changing directions, as tennis and soccer players often do. When your knee is bent too far, you lose power and compromise stability in your knee. When your heel is raised, it forces your calf muscles to do more work. (For more on this topic go to chapter 14, "Running with Shoes.")

   B. At some height, you will begin to lose power. What height is that?

   C. Rest when you are ready to move on.

6. Return to the same configuration and continue experimenting with where you can get more power in sliding the garage door. Here are some possible explorations:

   A. Turn your foot out 25 degrees and see how pushing this way affects your ankle, knee, and hip differently. Even your spine will be affected. Repeat a few times.

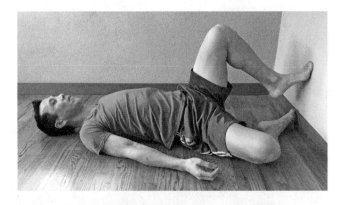

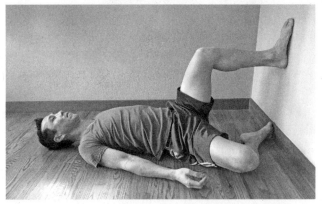

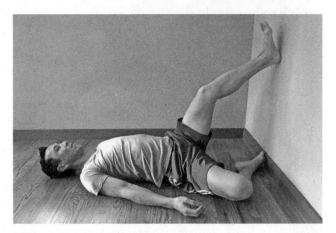

Sliding the imaginary door using 3 different positions for the front foot.

B. Turn your foot out 45 degrees and continue, observing the effects. Repeat a few times.

C. Place your foot so that the toes point directly at the ceiling. Repeat a few times as you compare the effects.

D. Turn your foot in 25 degrees and compare the effects.

E. Turn your foot in 45 degrees and compare. After repeating a few times, rest.

F. Note that each different angle for your foot will have a marked effect on how you use not only your left leg, but your entire body. As you probably observed, you gain more or less power depending on the direction in which your toes point. Your knee also feels more or less stable, depending on the direction. Turning your foot too far outward tends to result in less power and more undue torsion on your knee. Yet many people walk and run in this fashion due to what are conventionally called muscle imbalances, and what could be more appropriately thought of as biases in how they use their feet, legs, pelvis, and back.

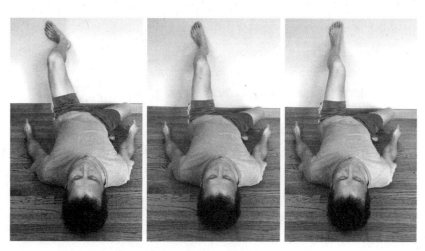

Right to left: neutral to extreme external rotation.

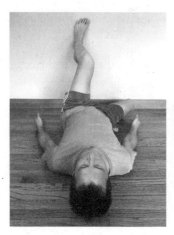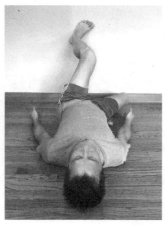

Left to right: minor and extreme internal rotation.

7. Choose any angle in which to point your foot, and this time, as you push the garage door, simultaneously spiral your foot outward (laterally). It is as if you are trying to screw your foot into the wall.

   A. Try this a few times, noticing the effect on your hip.

   B. Screw your foot in the other direction, noticing the difference.

   C. Rest.

8. Repeat each step on the other side. When you are finished, stand up and throw an imaginary ball a few times, noticing how you use your front leg. Walk and notice how your walking has changed.

Lesson 5
Flexing/Extending While
Throwing in Sitting[6]

Starting Position: Sit on the right corner of a chair, medium-height stool, or rectangular table such that your left foot points directly forward and your

---

[6] This lesson is closely related to Lesson 3, "Flexing/Extending While Throwing," and Lesson 9, "Reaching Up While Throwing."

right leg is a little behind you and out to the side.[7] Your right buttock will be off the chair or stool. Your right leg should be far enough behind so that your heel is off the floor.

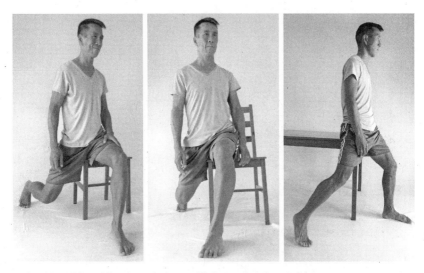

Left and middle: sitting in a chair or a high stool; right: a table.

1. Begin to rotate the right foot a little inward (medially) and then return to neutral.

   A. Your knee will begin to sink toward the midline as you rotate. Which toes and metatarsals are more involved? If you feel intense stretching in any of your toes, stop and put some books under your rear end so that you are sitting a little higher.

   B. Go back and forth, noticing the movement of your opposite foot and opposite leg. How does the weight shift on your opposite foot? How does it shift on your buttock?

   C. If it's comfortable to do so, rotate a little farther each time. You will feel your right knee moving closer to the midline.

---

[7] A high stool or table will be more appropriate for those who have long legs.

D. Is the right side of your pelvis moving?

E. Rest after a few trials.

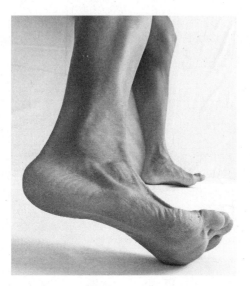

Close-up of right foot as it rotates inward
(medially).

2. Resume the previous movement. When you are at full rotation
with your back foot, gently push backward with your big toe and/or
second toe.

A. Try this a few times, then pause.

B. Now push with the ball of your foot, thereby extending the joint
where your big toe connects. What's the difference between
pushing with your toe(s) and with the ball of your foot?

C. As you push, notice how the weight shifts on your front foot.
Are you leaning forward when you reach your limit of rotating?
How far are your shoulders rotated?

D. Pause. Now begin to push backward with your front foot at the
same time that you push forward with the ball of your back

foot. Including the front foot and leg will likely increase the rotation of your pelvis and spine.

E. What happens in your lower abdomen when you engage your front foot? Does it contract? Expand? What is happening with your right shoulder?

F. Go back and forth, making sure that you are pushing with both feet.

G. Rest when you are ready.

3. Resume rotating your back foot, and this time do not push with your front foot. You will feel the weight shifting to the outside of your front foot. Your knee will start to shift outward, away from your midline.

A. Notice how this alters the movement of your right hip. What's happening in your lower abdomen?

B. Alternate between engaging your front foot and not engaging it with each rotation. Notice how engaging your front foot leads to contracting your abdomen, and not engaging it leads to expanding your abdomen.

C. Rest in the middle of the chair or stool when you feel like it.

4. Return to sitting on the side of your chair or stool. Cross your wrists and interlace your fingers.

A. Raise your arms above your head and begin to straighten your elbows. It will look as if you are trying to cover your ears with your biceps.

B. Don't be forceful lifting your arms and straightening your elbows if your shoulders are not so flexible. Simply reach gently upward with your hands.

C. With your arms in this position, begin to push with the ball of your back foot. Continue reaching upward with your arms at the same time and make sure you are not leaning forward at the end of your rotation.

D. For now, don't push back with your front foot. Simply allow the weight to shift on your front foot and your front knee to tilt outward.

E. Notice the expansion in your lower belly and in your chest. You may feel your back and hip extending more than before.

F. Go back and forth a few times, then pause. Drop your arms, maintaining the configuration of your spine. Resume rotating on the ball of your back foot. Pay attention to how lifted your chest is and how much your lower belly expands as you reach your rotational limit. *Note that this movement will likely bring relief to your back if you are accustomed to spending your days hunched over an electronic device.*

G. Go back and forth a few times, then rest.

5. Cross your wrists, interlace your fingers, and bring your arms over your head. This time as you reach for the ceiling, rotate your body by activating both your front foot and back foot.

A. Notice how pushing backward with your front leg leads your lower belly to contract.

B. Alternate between pushing back with your front leg and letting it roll outward. Notice how pushing and not pushing changes what happens in your belly and chest as well as in the extension of your hip.

C. Go back and forth a few times, then drop your arms, maintaining the configuration of your spine and pelvis. Continue rotating and alternating between pushing back your front leg and not pushing back with it.

D. Rest in the middle of the chair whenever you are done exploring. Sense the differences between your two hips, the two sides of your belly, and the two sides of your chest.

6. Walk around a little and compare how different your hips feel from each other.

7. Repeat all the steps on the other side.

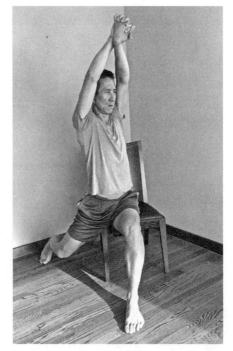

Rotating while reaching up with arms crossed.

Lesson 6
Screwing Foot into Floor[8]

Starting Position: Return to a throwing position with one foot in front and the other a little behind and out to the side. Rotate your pelvis and crush out the imaginary cigarette with the ball of your back foot. Feel free to

---

[8] Some of the motor concepts in this lesson will be further explored and reinforced in Lesson 17, "Reach and Roll on Your Back," Lesson 24, Rodin's Spiral," and Lesson 25, "Resistance as a Learning Tool."

change the position of your feet at any moment to improve your balance. Once you have found a stable position, leave your arms resting at your sides.

1. Lift all but the 1st metatarsal joint of your back foot.[9] Except for your big toe, lift all of your toes off the floor.

   A. Rotate your back foot internally (medially), noticing what's happening in your front foot. When you reach full internal (medial) rotation, pause and notice if you can still see your front ankle. If not, push your front hip backward: this action will simultaneously push your front knee backward.

   B. Once you've reached your rotational limit, rotate your back foot in the opposite direction, noticing how far you can go while still keeping all but your 1st metatarsal and big toe on the floor.

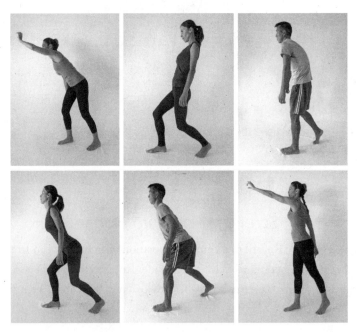

How are power, stability and comfort compromised in each of these examples?

---

[9] If you have sensitivities in your first metatarsal joint, start with the 2nd metatarsal or somewhere between the 1st and the 2nd.

C. Go back and forth slowly.

D. Exploring the movement with these constraints will increase the participation of parts of your feet and legs that may have been dormant for a long time. Rest frequently if you find your legs tiring quickly.

E. See to it that you are not leaning forward during the exploration. (If necessary, use a mirror to check.)

F. Finally, see if you can sink your chest back and downward almost as if to slouch—in order to keep your upper body directly over your pelvis. The sinking of your chest will help the tailbone to drop downward a little as your lower back to flattens, and all of this will force your legs to work more. (Note that while we are looking for a relatively flat spine in some of the "Throwing the Ball" lessons, a greater degree of curvature is healthy and normal when going about everyday life. Therefore, I do *not* recommend that you intentionally drop your tailbone or use any of the previously mentioned constraints except for exploratory purposes.)

G. Rest in standing, and notice if one arm feels longer than the other.

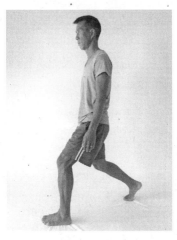

When you sink your chest, it will feel as if more weight has dropped into your legs.

2. Use adhesive tape to secure a few coins or a flat pebble under the 2nd metatarsal joint of your back foot. Repeat the previous steps, experimenting with rotating on the 2nd metatarsal of your back foot.

   A. Lift all of your toes and keep all but the 2nd metatarsal from touching the floor.

   B. When you are satisfied with exploring the 2nd metatarsal connection, shift the coins and your weight to the 3rd metatarsal and continue exploring. Rest whenever you feel like it.

   C. Play with this connection before shifting the coins and your weight to the 4th metatarsal.

   D. After playing with the 4th metatarsal, go on to the 5th metatarsal.

   E. As in Lesson 2, you will notice that as you change from 1st to 2nd, 2nd to 3rd, 3rd to 4th, and 4th to 5th, your leg rotates more externally and less internally.

3. Once again, explore rotating on different metatarsals, but this time allow all of your toes to touch the floor. Notice that when you *don't* lift your toes, the internal or external rotation of your hip will follow the *opposite* pattern as in the previous step: when you switch from 1st to 2nd, 2nd to 3rd, 3rd to 4th, and 4th to 5th, your leg will rotate more internally and less externally.[10] Rest after exploring each metatarsal.

4. Rest in standing and notice how one leg is more rooted into the floor. One arm will probably feel much longer as well.

5. Take a walk and notice how clearly your right foot rolls over the floor. The two sides of your body probably feel very different from each other.

6. Repeat as many steps as you want on the other side. When you are finished, go for a short walk or run to enjoy the increased clarity in your striding.

---

[10] We will reinforce the connection between the 4th and 5th metatarsal, hip extension, and internal rotation in Lesson 24, "Rodin's Spiral," and Lesson 25, "Resistance as a Learning Tool."

A final note: As you can see from the previous explorations, the range of internal or external (medial or lateral) rotation of your back hip depends not only on which metatarsal acts as the pivot point, but whether or not your toes are lifting off the floor. The relationship can be thought of as follows:

When you lift the toes of your back foot (as we did in Lesson 2, "Screwing Foot into Wall"): the range of internal rotation for your hip *decreases* as your balance point moves toward the outside of your back foot.

When you don't lift the toes of your back foot: the range of internal rotation for your hip *increases* as your balance point moves toward the outside of your back foot.

We will return to this relationship between the toes, metatarsals, and internal and external rotation of the hip in Lesson 24, "Rodin's Spiral."

Lesson 7 (Advanced)[11]
Downward Spiral[12]

Starting Position: Throw an imaginary ball with either hand, making sure that your opposite foot is forward. Freeze at the end of your throw, then leave your arms resting at your sides.

1. Begin to crush out the cigarette with the 4th and 5th metatarsals of your back foot—essentially, the outer part of the ball of your foot. (Note that there is no need to lift your toes in this lesson.)

    A. Go back and forth a few times and note once again how being on the outside of the back foot allows you to rotate farther.

    B. Rest in standing. Your two feet will likely feel quite different from each other.

---

[11] Be particularly careful with steps 3, 4, and 5 if you have any knee or foot issues. As I mentioned earlier, it's important to approach the advanced lessons cautiously since they will make demands on parts of your body that may have been dormant for a long time. To reduce your risk of injury: (1) be prepared to stop frequently and spread the lesson over days, weeks, or even months; (2) avoid any movements that result in a feeling of intense stretching (if you feel intense stretching in any part of yourself, you are probably going *way* too far); (3) consider skipping any part that feels risky.

[12] Rest assured that this downward spiral is followed by an upward one!

2. Repeat the last step as you sink your chest back and downward—almost as if to slouch. As your chest sinks, allow your tailbone to drop downward a little. You will feel your lower back flattening. Once again, this action will make you feel heavier.

   A. Notice how much more your legs must work when your chest is slightly sunken.

   B. Go back and forth a few times, then rest.

   C. Walk around to sense the changes in your gait. The way you roll off your right foot should feel quite different from the way you roll off your left. You may feel your right hip extending more as you walk.

3. Note that steps 3, 4, and 5 are on a higher order of difficulty. If you have any knee or foot issues, skip to step 6. Otherwise, proceed cautiously.

   A. In order to protect your heel on this next step, you may want to wear a very thin-soled shoe with a very flexible sole, or place a thin piece of sticky foam or a yoga mat under your front foot.

   B. Lift the entire ball of your front foot such that only your heel is in contact with the floor. Begin to rotate both feet simultaneously so that the front foot turns out and the back foot turns in. (For now, allow the weight on your back foot to migrate to any metatarsal it wants to as you crush out the cigarette.)

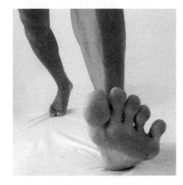

Lift the ball of your front foot.

   C. Go slowly and notice that your body rotates much farther when you pivot on the heel of your front foot. Notice also that it's more difficult to control the movement.

D. As you rotate farther, notice how the weight transfers to the *outside* of the ball of your back foot—where the 4th and 5th metatarsals reside. This should happen naturally, serving the dual purpose of protecting your back knee while allowing you to rotate farther and more easily.

E. Gradually allow the movement to get larger. Your front foot may rotate so far that its entire outside edge touches the floor. Don't be discouraged if you find yourself losing your balance along the way. This is a fairly tricky motion and it will likely take some time to become more proficient. Safety is more important than achievement; don't feel obligated to rotate as far as you can.

F. Rest whenever you want to.

4. Resume the previous step and notice if you are holding your breath.

A. Don't worry too much about making a large movement. Mainly, see if you can rotate without holding your breath or clenching your jaw. Even if the rotation is small, there are enormous benefits. It's generally better to stay small and move with finesse than to make the movement large but lose control in the process.

B. Rest whenever you want to.

5. Resume the previous step. If you haven't already, see if you can rotate far enough such that the outside edge of your front foot is on the floor.

A. Go back and forth a few times slowly. Notice the moments that you start to hold your breath.

B. The next time the entire edge of your front foot is on the floor, begin to lower your rear end a little. As you go lower, your back knee will begin to fold under you. You will feel certain toes stretching. If you feel an intense stretch in your toes or in the sole of your foot, you have gone too far.

C. Only lower yourself an inch or so and then come back up. Move slowly and with control. Your legs and feet will feel very awake.

D. Rest.

6. Repeat the previous step, but this time sink your rear end another inch toward the floor.

A. Go back and forth two or three times, each time sinking an inch farther.

B. If you are doing this for the first time, don't go too low. I don't recommend sinking too far until you've done this lesson several times and your body has gotten used to this movement.

C. Rest.

7. Return to throwing the ball. Notice if the movement feels more stable and powerful. Walk around and feel the differences in your gait.

8. Repeat each step with the opposite leg forward. When you are finished, walk and see what effect the lesson has on your chest and shoulders. Notice how different your feet feel as you walk.

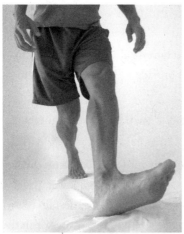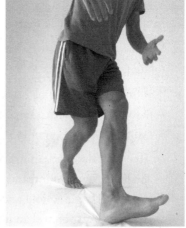

As you rotate, transfer your weight toward the outside of your back foot— somewhere around the 4th and 5th metatarsals.

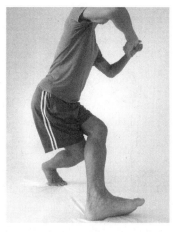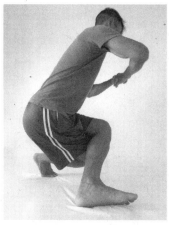

As you lower your rear end, your back knee will fold under your front leg.

Lesson 8
Stabilizing Your Front Leg
While Throwing

Starting Position: Return to the stance for throwing your imaginary ball. Be ready to adjust your stance, for example, widening or narrowing it, if it helps you maintain your balance. Leave your arms resting at your sides.

1. Lift all the toes of your front foot high in the air and see to it that you are not leaning forward. Now begin to evert your front foot—that is, lift the outside edge of your front foot. The little toe will begin to rise a little and the big toe will sink a little. Notice how the 1st metatarsal joint of your front foot begins to press more into the ground. Also notice how your front knee collapses a little inward (to the right).

A. With your front foot in this position, begin to slowly rotate on the ball of your back foot. (In this lesson we won't be focusing on the metatarsals of the back foot.) This will probably feel like a balancing act in the beginning, so go slowly and feel free to reposition either or both feet. I recommend *not* making large movements for now. If you feel *any* tenderness in your front knee, stop *immediately* and skip to step 5.

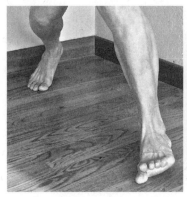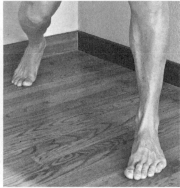

Notice the difference between the everted foot (left) and the slightly inverted foot (right).

B. Notice how the outside edge of your front foot wants to drop. See to it that your front foot stays strongly everted—that is, the outside edge stays up in the air. The simple act of maintaining eversion in your front foot will keep your knee collapsed inward. It will also limit the rotation of your pelvis.

C. Go back and forth once or twice, then rest.

2. Repeat step 1, but this time freeze at the end of your rotation with the outside edge of your front foot still lifted. Allow the outside edge of your front foot to return to the floor.

A. As the weight shifts toward the outside of your front foot, you will feel your pelvis simultaneously rotating farther.

B. Shift your weight back and forth on your front foot from the inside to the outside and back, and feel how your pelvis rotates in one direction, then the other, depending on where your weight is shifting. Also notice how your shoulders rotate in synchrony with your pelvis.

C. Finally notice how your front knee moves side to side, from a collapsed position to a more stable position and back.

D. Rest whenever you feel like it.

3. Repeat step 2 and notice that as you shift the weight from the inside to the outside of your front foot, your front knee will tend to spiral outward and backward (counterclockwise if it's your left foot, clockwise if it's your right foot).

   A. The farther outward your knee travels, the more you will feel the intrinsic muscles of the foot activating and the arch rising in your foot. The spiraling motion of your front tibia and knee, along with the subsequent rising of the arch, help to protect your knee while increasing rotational force.

   B. Go back and forth a few times, experimenting with the spiraling motion of your front knee. Make the spirals gradually bigger and then gradually smaller before resting.

4. Return to your throwing position. If you haven't already, begin to sink your chest inward and downward, going into a slight slouch. Once again, the sinking of your chest will lead your tailbone to drop downward a little, and your lower back to flatten.

   A. Begin to rotate again, allowing your weight to shift to the outside of your front foot.

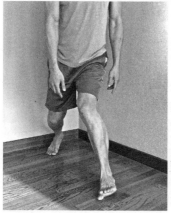 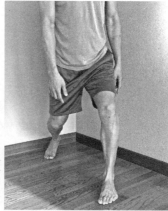

Everting your front foot (left) will significantly change the movement of your pelvis and spine. Compare everting the front foot to allowing the weight on that foot to spiral outward (right).

B. Rotating with your chest sunken this way tends to increase the rotation of your pelvis.

C. Go back and forth, comparing what it's like to rotate with your chest in and with it out. Rest whenever you want to.

5. Repeat the previous step, and this time pay attention to the movement of your front knee.

A. When your chest is sunk in this fashion, your pelvis will likely rotate farther and your knee will consequently spiral outward and backward. (If your left knee is forward, it will spiral in a counterclockwise direction. If your right knee is forward, it will spiral in a clockwise direction.)

B. When your chest isn't sunken, your pelvis will likely rotate less and your knee will probably not move backward. In fact, if you do the opposite and protrude your chest, there will be a tendency to stand up taller at the end of your rotation.

C. Experiment with sinking your chest and protruding it, and see how it affects different aspects of your rotation.

D. We will return to how the positioning of the spine affects rotation in the next lesson.

E. Rest.

6. Walk around and feel the differences between your two sides.

7. Repeat all the steps on the other side.

Lesson 9
Reaching Up While Throwing[13]

Starting Position: Return to the familiar stance for throwing the imaginary ball. Leave your arms resting at your sides.

---

[13] This lesson continues some of the themes that are evident in Lesson 3, "Flexing/Extending While Throwing," and Lesson 5, "Flexing/Extending While Throwing in Sitting." It is also a useful precursor to Lesson 15, "Reaching Up."

1. Sink your chest inward and downward until you feel your lower back is relatively flat. Once again, the sinking of your chest will lead your tailbone to drop downward a little and your lower back to flatten. Your legs will have to work more while your lower back will probably feel relieved.

   A. Begin to rotate on your back foot as if to crush out a cigarette.

   B. Allow your weight to shift to the outside of your front foot.

   C. Rotating with your chest sunken this way tends to increase the rotation of your pelvis.

   D. Go back and forth, comparing what it's like to rotate with your chest in and chest out. Rest whenever you want to.

2. Repeat the previous step, and this time pay attention to the movement of your front knee.

   A. As we discovered in Lesson 8, when your chest has sunk in this fashion, your pelvis will likely rotate farther and your front knee will consequently spiral outward and backward. (If your left knee is forward, it will spiral in a counterclockwise direction; If your right knee is forward, it will spiral in a clockwise direction.)

   B. When your chest isn't sunken, your pelvis will likely rotate less and your knee will probably not move backward.

   C. Experiment with sinking the center of your chest more and sinking it less. Notice how each change increases or reduces the spiraling of your front knee, the rotating of your pelvis, and the extending of your back hip.

   D. Rest.

3. Return to your throwing position, but this time cross your arms and interlace your fingers. Lift your arms above your head and begin to straighten your elbows by reaching upward, as if you wanted to squeeze your ears with your arms. In this configuration, you will feel the center of your chest rising instead of sinking.

   A. Begin to rotate on your back foot.

   B. Go back and forth a few times, then pause.

C. Drop your arms, keeping your spine in the same configuration. Notice how much your chest continues to lift.

D. Resume rotating on your back foot.

E. Go back and forth a few times, then rest.

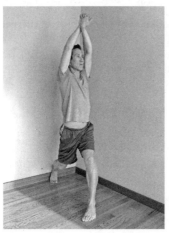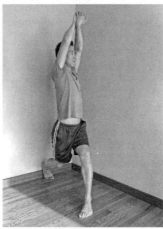

Crossing arms and reaching up as you rotate.

4. Resume the previous step with arms down. This time alternate once with your chest rising and once with your chest sinking.

A. Notice the difference between having your chest rise and having it sink. You will feel the difference, not only in your spine, but in how you use your legs and feet.

B. When you are satisfied with comparing the differences, rest.

5. In standing, notice how different your two legs feel from each other. Your shoulders and arms will probably also feel quite different from each other as well. With these types of explorations, a neuromuscular change will occur throughout your entire body, affecting the muscle tonus of the entire right and left sides differently. If you pay close attention, you will notice that the two sides

of your face feel different. Close your eyes and sense which side of your face feels more relaxed. Which side feels more alive? Take a walk and enjoy the differences.

6. Repeat each step with the opposite foot forward.

Lessons 10–17

Lesson 10
Standing Tall Without Trying to Stand Tall

Preliminary Experiment: Walk up a flight of stairs and feel how much effort it requires and which muscles are getting tired. Do it a few times, testing what happens when you look down at your feet compared to looking straight forward. Compare leaning forward more to leaning forward less. After getting a sense of how different ways of climbing stairs affect your sense of effort, try the following lesson.

Starting Position: Lie on your stomach, turn your head to the right, and place your hands palm down, under your cheek, with the right hand on top. Lift your head once. On a scale of 1 to 10, how heavy is it?

1. Imagine your left cheek is glued to the back of your right hand. Lift your head and right arm at the same time. See to it that your elbow and hand stay at the same height. Go up and down, feeling the parts of your back that start to get activated. Notice if you feel your buttocks contracting. Continue two or three times very slowly—go slowly enough that it takes five seconds to reach the top and five to reach the bottom. Rest with your head turned to the left.

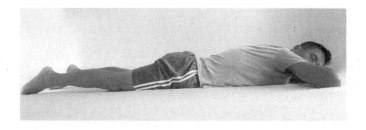

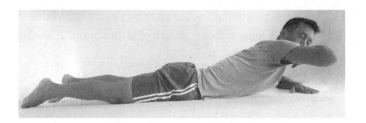

2. Turn your head back to the right, and keeping your left leg straight, begin to lift your left foot in the air. Feel the muscles in your buttocks and back that begin to get activated as your foot goes higher. Move your foot straight toward the ceiling and then try different angles—for example, toward the ceiling and to the right a few degrees. Feel how lifting your foot in different angles affects the movement of your pelvis and back differently. Performing each variation will activate different muscles all the way up your spine. Rest with your head turned to the left.

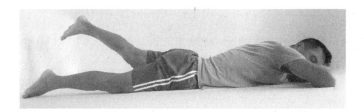

3. Return to having your head turned to the right. Lift your head, right arm, and left foot all at the same time. Does your head feel lighter? When any part of your body feels heavy, it is often because other parts are not activated. In this case, activating parts of your lower back and even your buttock help to lift your head.

   A. Notice if you are tightening your abs, and note that doing so makes the movement more difficult. Experiment with tightening your abs and increasing the contractions with each lift to see what happens.

B. Now do the opposite: begin to inflate your abdominal region like a balloon, which will push it into the floor. Does this make the movement easier? Repeat a few times and rest.

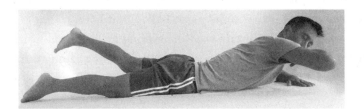

4. Return to the previous position. This time lift your right foot while lifting your head and right arm. How is this in comparison to doing it with your left foot? Repeat a few times.

5. Repeat steps 1 to 4 in the opposite configuration (with your head turned to the left, and your left hand on top of the right).

6. Finally, place your forehead on your hands (either hand on top) and lift your head and both arms together. Explore a few times, noticing the activation of muscles all the way down to your buttocks. Even your feet will move a little.

   A. Now try the movement while lifting both feet at the same time. Which lifts higher, your head or your feet?

   B. As a variation, try it a few times with your chin resting on your right hand. Lift your right arm, head, and right foot at the same time. Repeat a few times and then try lifting your right arm, head, and left foot at the same time. Repeat a few times and then rest before trying it with your left arm.

   C. With your chin on both hands, lift your head, arms, and both legs. Repeat a few times, sensing which elbow and which foot lift higher. Rest.

   D. Go back to having your head turned to the right. Lift it slowly once or twice to see if it's gotten lighter. On a scale of 1 to 10, how heavy is it now?

7. When you stand, notice how tall and erect you are. Climb a flight of stairs or walk up a hill with this tallness. Notice how much easier it is to climb when you are standing tall, rather than leaning forward. I've found that the difference is quite dramatic. I play with hills regularly, and it never ceases to amaze me that certain ways of carrying my head and lifting upward give me so much more power. It's like adding turbo-charge to my stride.

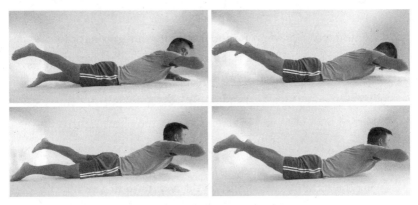

Step 4 (upper left), 6a (upper right), 6b (bottom left), 6c (bottom right).

Lesson 11
Lift Your Knees (On Your Back, Raising Your Knee toward Your Chest and the Ceiling)

Starting Position: Lie on your back with both legs bent and both feet standing on the floor.

1. Begin to lift your right knee up toward your chest (allow your leg to stay bent). How easy is it to move your right knee? What are you doing with your left leg? Go back and forth a few times slowly, in order to feel which muscles you are using. Pause. Now begin to reach your right knee forward toward the ceiling. Does

it move at all? Is it even possible to move your knee in this direction? Pause.

A. Now press your left foot into the floor as you lift your right knee toward the ceiling. Push with enough force to lift your butt off the floor. Notice how the pressing into your left foot varies the ease or difficulty of moving your right knee. Go back and forth a few times.

B. As you press with your left foot, begin to move your knee toward your chest. Feel how much easier it is to lift your knee in this direction compared to when you don't press with your foot. Vary the amount that you press with your left foot and notice how this makes the right knee easier or harder to move. Go back and forth several times slowly. Rest with your legs long.

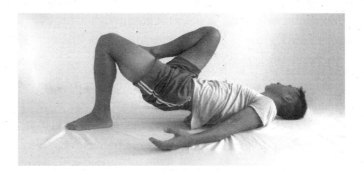

2. Bend your knees again and repeat the last step, but this time notice how close your left heel is to your buttocks.

A. Begin to vary that distance, noticing how it affects the lifting of your right knee toward your chest. Do you get more power when you place your left foot closer or farther away from your buttocks?

B. Begin to reach your right knee forward, toward the ceiling. Notice how varying the location of your left foot affects the ease or difficulty in reaching with the opposite knee. Pause.

3. Now instead of pressing with your left foot, lift it a tiny bit off the floor and try reaching your right knee forward toward the ceiling again. Once again, it might feel quite impossible to move it.

   A. With your left foot still off the floor, begin to bring your right knee toward your chest. How easy is it to move your knee in this direction? Which muscles are exerting more effort?

   B. Many people lift their legs somewhat independently of the rest of their body when walking or running. Yet, as you are probably noticing now, lifting one knee without pushing back with the opposite leg dramatically decreases your power.[14] In a moment you will discover how involving the upper body further adds to your power. Rest.

4. Hold the front of your right knee with your left hand. Get a good grip (your thumb should be touching your index finger, and all fingers should be pointing to the right). Begin to pull your knee up toward your left shoulder. What are you doing with your left leg?

   A. Notice that when you pull your knee, your shoulder moves toward it at the same time. Which way does your head want to roll? (Remember, if your eyes lock on a target, it will likely freeze your neck muscles and stop your head from moving freely.)

   B. Play with this movement for a while, searching for what your head really wants to do. Close your eyes and see if it helps to free your neck.

---

[14] In reality the trajectory of each knee in walking is determined by a far more complex process involving more than just the "pushing back" action of the opposite leg. Lesson 13, "Behind Your Behind," along with Lessons 22 and 23 from the "Metatarsals to Metacarpals" series, can give you a deeper sense of how everything going on behind your back crucially affects what's going on in front. Note that Nicholas Romanov of the *Pose Method of Running* (Coral Gables, FL: Pose Method Publishing, 2004) and Danny Dreyer and Katherine Dreyer of *ChiRunning: A Revolutionary Approach to Effortless, Injury-Free Running* (New York: Simon & Schuster, 2004) also address this issue, though in a different manner.

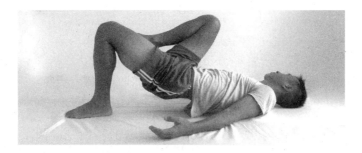

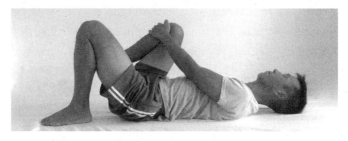

5. Go back to the same configuration (holding your right knee with your left hand) and continue pulling your knee toward your shoulder and allow your shoulder to move toward your knee.

A. Begin pushing with your left foot into the floor, and notice how much more your opposite knee lifts—both toward your shoulder and toward the ceiling.

B. Allow your head to roll to the side if it feels more comfortable. Repeat the entire movement a few times slowly and then rest.

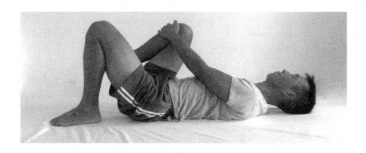

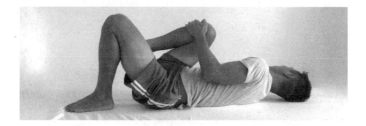

6. Leave your arms at your sides and continue pushing with your left foot into the floor. This time, reach your knee closer and closer to the ceiling. You will be pushing with quite a bit of force with your left leg. Do you feel the muscles working in your left buttock?

   A. Feel how connected your right knee is to the extension of your left hip (see the photos below).

   B. Experiment with placing your left foot in closer or farther away from your buttocks.

   C. Return to holding your right knee with your left hand. Once again, bring your knee toward your shoulder and your shoulder toward

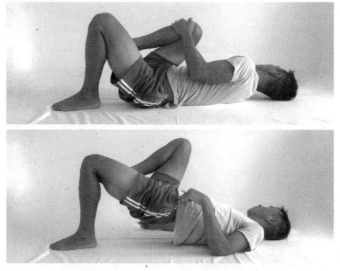

Extending either hip (the left hip in both examples) affects the lifting and thrusting of the opposite knee.

your knee. Compare the difference in how your body moves now that you are holding your knee, and notice how the movement of your trunk affects the movement of your knee. Rest.

7. Bend your knees and hold your right knee with your left hand. This time lift your head, shoulders, and upper back off the floor before you begin (like doing a partial sit-up, your chest will come toward the ceiling).

   A. Begin to push your knee forward toward the ceiling. Go forward toward the ceiling and back down a few times. You will notice that two things happen: (1) your knee doesn't move as far as before; and (2) the movement is much more effortful.

   B. Lifting your shoulders and head has pushed your center of gravity down into your hips, making it much more difficult to extend your left hip. Your left leg now has much more weight to push against. Note that this configuration is a simulation of what happens when you lean too far forward when running.[15]

8. After you have rested, repeat each step on the other side.

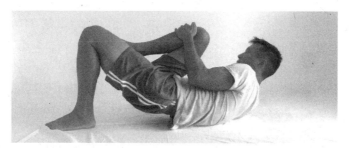

Leaning too far forward or holding your abdominals too tightly while running can reduce the power of your stride. Note in the photo how curving forward makes it harder for me to extend my left hip.

---

[15] As we shall see in Lesson 24, "Rodin's Spiral," and Lesson 25, "Resistance as a Learning Tool," a similar difficulty occurs in boxing when a boxer attempts to throw an uppercut while leaning forward at the same time. For a good description of this, see Precision Striking, "Boxer Uppercut Tips: 5 Common Errors, Part 1 of 3," YouTube, October 11, 2017, https://youtu.be/GBRRy905Q2Q.

Lesson 12 (Advanced)[16]
Mobilizing Your Rib Cage

Starting Position: Lie on your back and bend your knees so that your feet are flat on the floor. Hold your left knee with your right hand. Place your left hand on the outside edge of your left knee and begin to slide it down your shin toward your left foot.

1. Go slowly, sliding your hand a few inches and then sliding back to the knee. Each time, slide your hand a little farther. Notice that as your hand gets closer to your foot, the left side of your rib cage begins to bend like an accordion. You may feel your head rolling to the left or sliding such that the top of your head comes a little closer to the floor.

   A. Go back and forth a few times, slowly and gently, sensing how your back and neck respond. Notice if you are unintentionally restricting the movement of your neck. If you feel tension building up, start over and slow down your movements, and begin to experiment with rolling, sliding, and tilting your head in different directions as you reach, seeing which directions decrease tension and which ones increase it.

   B. Rest.

2. Repeat the previous step and continue sliding your hand farther until you reach the outside edge of your left foot. (If you feel increasing tension and strain in your neck as you reach, I recommend you stop and continue this lesson on another day.)

   A. Once you reach the outside edge, slide your hand underneath to hold the bottom of your foot. If you have to strain to hold the bottom of your foot, then hold your ankle instead.

---

[16] Perhaps even more than with other lessons, advanced lessons should be approached with great care and attention since any given step may make demands on parts of your body that have been dormant for a long time. To reduce your risk of injury: (1) be prepared to stop frequently and spread the lesson over days, weeks, or even months; (2) avoid any movements that result in a feeling of intense stretching: if you feel intense stretching in any part of yourself, you are probably going *way* too far; (3) consider skipping any part that feels risky.

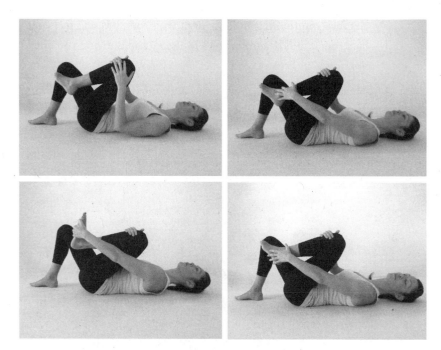

From top left clockwise to bottom left: Sliding the left hand toward the bottom of the foot.

    B. Make sure to find a position for your head that allows your neck to be as comfortable as possible.

    C. Let go of your foot and slide your hand back to your knee.

    D. Continue sliding your hand back and forth from your knee the bottom of your foot (or your ankle, if it's a strain to reach your foot), sensing how your rib cage, neck, and head respond. Repeat a few times, then rest.

3. Once again, slide your hand and hold the bottom of your left foot (or ankle). Begin to move your foot toward the ceiling.

    A. As your foot moves toward the ceiling, you will feel muscles in your left leg becoming very active. Your hamstrings will begin to elongate. Start with a small movement.

B. Because your hand is holding onto your foot, you will feel your back, neck, and head moving. Go *slowly* and notice if you are holding your breath.

C. Move your leg up and down easily and smoothly, gradually making the movement larger. Rest after going up and down a few times.

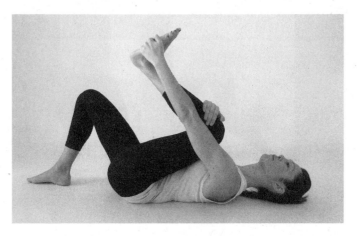

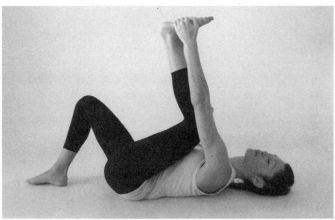

4. Return to the same configuration, but this time hold the back of your head with your right hand. Begin to lift your left foot and head at the same time, slowly. Try turning your head in different

directions as you lift to see which is more comfortable. Explore the simultaneous lifting of your head and foot several times, resting whenever you want. Notice how differently your trunk moves when you are holding your head and lifting it at the same time.

5. Now try holding the inside of your left foot with your right hand and the back of your head with your left hand. Lift your foot and head and notice how differently your leg and entire spine move compared to when you were in the previous configuration. Go up and down several times, resting whenever you want.

6. Take a full rest with your arms and legs long. Notice how different the two sides of your body feel. Which leg and arm feel longer? Which side of your face feels longer?

7. Repeat steps 1 to 5 on the other side, then rest and notice if the two sides feel less different than before.

8. Bring your knees over your chest, reach between your legs, and hold the inside arch of your right foot with your right hand (the palm of your hand should be against the arch of your foot), and the inside arch of your left foot with your left hand. Begin to lift your feet toward the ceiling, moving them apart as they rise.

   A. Raise your feet and lower them, allowing your head to roll, tilt, or slide on the floor in any way that reduces tension and makes the movement easier. As your feet go up and farther apart, you may feel your chin wanting to move away from your chest. In other words, the back of your head may spontaneously begin sliding toward the area between your shoulders.

   B. Repeat a few times, then rest.

9. Repeat the previous step, but this time lift your head up and keep it up as you lift your feet.

   A. How is the movement different when you lift your head? What is happening in your shoulders and neck? Can you explore the movement without tensing up your shoulders or locking your elbows?

B. Make sure you are not straining your neck. If you feel any strain or fatigue in your neck, stop and rest before moving on to the next step.

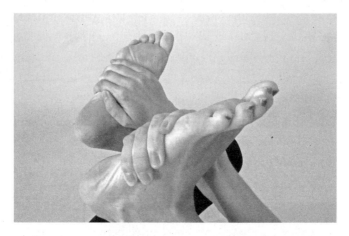

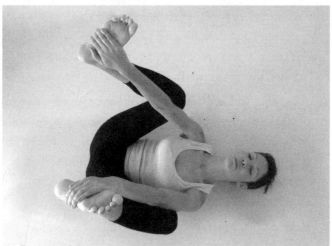

10. Reach between your legs again, but this time hold the outside of each foot: your right palm is against the dorsal side your right foot (where your shoelaces would be if you were wearing shoes) and your fingers wrap around the outside edge of the right foot; the left hand

does the same on the left foot. Lift the feet several times toward the ceiling. Try it without lifting your head for a few trials before doing it while you lift your head. Compare the differences. Rest.

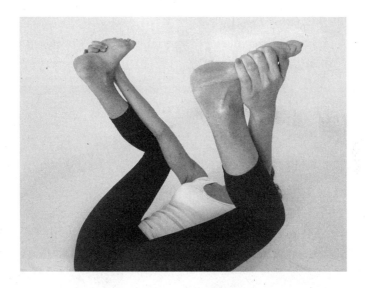

11. Hold the front of your left knee with your left hand and the arch of your left foot with your right hand. Bring your knee toward your chest and your head toward your knee. Experiment with aiming your knee at different parts of your chest on both your left and right side.

   A. Now switch your hands so that your right hand is on your left knee and your left hand reaches around the outside of your leg to hold the outside of your left foot. Bring your knee toward your chest and your head toward your knee at the same time.

   B. Go back and forth, switching hands to compare the difference in how your left hip moves. Also notice how your rib cage and shoulders move. Rest.

12. Hold your left knee with your right hand and the outside of your left foot with your left hand. Begin to make circles with your left

foot—as if you were washing an imaginary window with the sole of your foot. Go slowly and see if you can make increasingly accurate circles (rather than ovals). You have the option of lifting your head and watching your foot move, or leaving it on the floor and allowing it to roll, tilt, or slide.

   A. If you feel even the *slightest* strain in your neck, it means you have gone too far.

   B. After a few repetitions, change directions of the circles. Make sure you rest whenever you need to.

13. Repeat steps 11 and 12 on the other side.

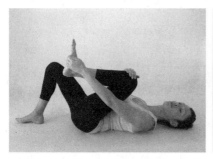 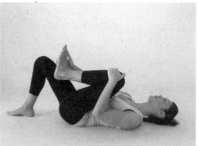

Left: circles with the right hand to the left foot; Right: with the left hand to the left foot.

14. Advanced Step 1: Reach between your legs and hold the insides of your arches with your hands. Begin to reach the sole of your left foot toward the ceiling as your right knee reaches toward the floor. Let your head roll gently on the floor.

   A. Once your right knee touches (your left leg will be relatively straight), reverse the movement until your right leg is relatively straight and your left knee is touching the ground.

   B. Go back and forth slowly. Go slowly and see how well you can control the movement. The more control you have, the softer the landing for either knee.

15. Advanced Step 2: Repeat step 14, but this time lift your head and keep your head off the floor. Be careful not to strain your neck. If your head feels very heavy from the outset, it's probably better to skip this step. (Note that the feeling of heaviness doesn't necessarily mean you have a weak neck. The relative heaviness or lightness of your head is more closely related to how you are organizing your lumbar spine and rib cage.)

16. Optional Test: try steps 8, 9, or 10 to see if they have gotten easier.

17. Stand up and notice how full your breath has become and how light your shoulders and chest feel. Do you feel more rooted into your legs? Do you feel taller? Walk and see if your steps feel more fluid and stable.

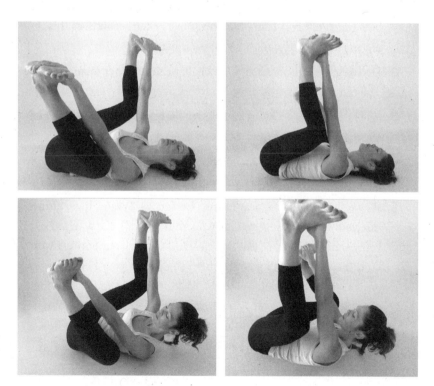

Above: rolling while keeping the head on the floor; below: rolling while lifting the head.

Lesson 13
Behind Your Behind

This lesson, inspired in part by one of the *shuaijiao* drills I learned from Master Li and Master Ge, has helped me to better understand that what goes on behind me affects everything that goes on in front.[17] There are two parts to this lesson. In part 1, you will lift your knees higher by focusing on lifting your knees higher. In part 2, you will discover that by bringing your attention to the motion of each foot as it moves behind you, your knees will lift with a surprising combination of ease and power.

PART 1: DRIVING YOUR KNEES BY TRYING TO DRIVE YOUR KNEES

Starting Position: Standing (in preparation for walking uphill).

1. Find a sizeable hill and begin running up. Try to go quickly and see how much effort it takes. Stop after five or ten seconds, as this is not meant to be a workout.

2. Go back to the bottom and use chalk or some other means to measure out approximately six-inch intervals.

3. As you begin to walk, lift your knees higher and higher—exaggerate your motion to bring your knees very high.

4. Notice how your arms and shoulders start to get more involved as your knees go higher. Are you looking down at your feet?

5. As we shall see in the next lesson (Lesson 14, "Water Jugs, Furniture, and Other Things to Carry on Your Head"), the way you use your Achilles tendons, calf muscles, and indeed your entire lower body is inextricably linked to what you do with your head. For now, notice what's happening with the back of your neck. Is it curving more or less than usual? Is it bending forward? If you are not doing so already, look straight ahead into the distance rather than down. Your gaze will influence the elongation of your spine.

---

[17] *Shuaijiao* is a millennia-old grappling art bearing some resemblance to both Mongolian wrestling and Judo.

6. Start to stride easily, but do not try to cover a lot of ground. Intentionally drive your knees upward as if you are trying to stride over a barrier. This way you will be traveling more upward than forward. Again, check the back of your neck to see if it is long and straight. Make sure you are looking into the distance and not downward.

7. See if you can cover no more than six inches per stride.

8. Do this for about one minute, then walk to the bottom of the hill and rest for a few minutes before continuing.

PART 2: DRIVING YOUR KNEES WITHOUT TRYING TO DRIVE THEM

Starting Position: Standing (in preparation for walking uphill).

1. Begin walking up the hill again, but this time focus on how each foot travels behind you. Being unaware of what's happening behind their backs and focusing too heavily on driving their knees forward and up, many people inadvertently truncate the full motion of the foot as it travels behind their body. Unfortunately, such truncation decreases propulsive power in their stride and actually prevents the knees from driving with as much power.

    A. Which heel travels closer to your buttocks?

    B. Stop. Now step forward with your left foot and freeze, leaving your right foot behind you, but with the ball of the right foot still connected with the ground.

    C. Imagine having a small coin underneath the ball of your right foot. Forcefully shoot the coin backward as if you are attempting to hit something behind you. (If this image doesn't work for you, imagine that you have a piece of paper stuck on the ball of your foot and want to wipe it off by quickly sliding the foot backward.) If you allow your right leg to be loose, your right knee will automatically bend and shoot forward. The thrusting forward of your right knee will feel effortless.

    D. Step forward again with your left foot and continue the process of shooting the coin backward with the ball of your right foot.

E. Continue walking, each time shooting a coin from underneath your right foot.

F. You will notice that this action does something interesting to the trajectory of your right foot as it travels behind you. You will also notice that your right knee lifts higher as a result. Can you feel how the shooting of the coin thrusts your left shoulder forward?

G. After a while you can try shooting coins from beneath your left foot and notice how it affects the trajectory of your left foot, left knee, and right shoulder.

H. Now begin shooting coins with every step—that is, from under the right foot, then left, then right … back and forth.

I. Play with this movement for a short while, then rest.

2. Repeat the shooting of coins from under the right foot, but this time while jogging.

A. Notice how this affects the movement of your right foot and right knee. Notice also how it affects the movement of your left arm and left shoulder.

B. Play with this for a while before switching to shooting coins from under your left foot as you jog. How does switching sides affect the movement of your left foot, left knee, and right arm?

C. After exploring how shooting coins from the left foot affects your stride, begin shooting coins from underneath either foot with each stride. Stay focused on shooting the coins rather than trying to lift your knees or increase your speed. Notice how your knees lift easily and with relatively little effort. Does it feel easier to jog up the hill this way? Do you feel increased power in your stride even though you are probably exerting less effort than usual?

D. Simply by shooting the coins in an ever more relaxed manner, your knees will lift higher and you will find your stride lengthening. See if you can refrain from leaning forward, and instead, stay tall. Do *not* attempt to cover as much ground as possible. How does staying tall affect your stride? See if you feel your legs working differently than usual. Are you finding it easier to run uphill?

3. Rest whenever you want to.

4. Note that any of these explorations from this lesson can be repeated when climbing stairs. As you may have guessed, shooting coins from the balls of your feet also makes stair climbing easier. Furthermore, if you tend to trip while going up stairs, this lesson will quickly rectify this tendency.

Lesson 14
Water Jugs, Furniture, and
Other Things to Carry on Your Head[18]

Starting Position: Sit at the edge of a sturdy, armless chair (preferably with little or no cushioning so that you can really feel your sit bones on the chair) with your feet firmly planted on the floor. Make sure the chair is large enough such that your hips are at least as high as your knees, if not a little higher (for people with long legs, you will need a high stool). Close your eyes and use one index finger to touch the bony protuberance at the top of your neck—where your neck meets your skull. This is your occiput. Place your other index finger on the middle of your chin.

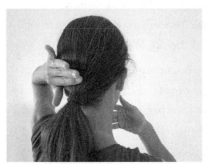
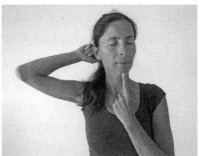

1. Begin to collapse the back of your neck so that your chin juts farther and farther forward. Your chest will also begin to collapse and you will begin to hunch. Most of us are doing some less exaggerated version of

---

[18] Lesson 20, "Making Your Head Lighter," provides a different perspective on some of the motor concepts that you will explore in this lesson.

this in daily life even though it may be causing us neck and back pain. Notice how the occiput begins to move down toward the ground as the chin moves forward and up. They move in opposite directions.

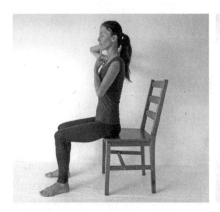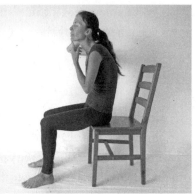

Left: When the *baihui* rises, the spine will tend to elongate. Right: Notice how Andreia's entire spine moves with the movement of her chin.

2. Now begin to do the opposite. Begin to lengthen the back of your neck such that your chin starts to come in toward your throat. You will feel your occiput start to rise. You will also feel some part of the top of your head reaching for the sky. Which part is it?

3. If you lengthen the back of the neck beyond a certain point, your head will start to tip so that your nose (and thus your face) ends up pointing downward. If you don't lengthen enough, your nose will be pointing a little upward.

   A. Go back and forth slowly and start to get a sense of the middle point, where the back of your neck is long and you feel effortlessly tall.

   B. Sense how, at this point, a certain part of your head reaches for the sky. You have just discovered a vital point on the top of your head. Bagua masters call this point the *baihui* (pronounced "bye-whey"), which in qigong and Traditional Chinese Medicine translates to the convergence of all yang meridians.

4. Repeat the previous steps, with your hands switched (if your right index finger was on your chin, place it on your occiput). If you use a mirror, you will notice that your head will naturally turn toward whichever hand you place in front.

5. Imagine a hook connected to your *baihui* being pulled gently toward the sky, as if you were a marionette.

6. Stand up and try walking while you collapse the back of your neck so that your chin begins to jut forward. Notice that the more you collapse your neck, the more your chest sinks in and the heavier your body feels. Now attempt to lengthen the back of your neck and notice how this feels in comparison. Lifting the top of your head actually helps to lift your rib cage. Thus, in lifting your *baihui*, you will likely feel not only more comfortable but lighter. You are beginning to tap into a critical technique used by Bagua masters, Olympic runners, and indeed millions of women around the world who transport everything from water and food to clothing and furniture on top of their heads.[19]

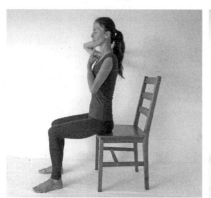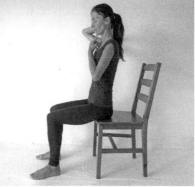

Baihui rising (left) compared to a slight forward tipping of the head (right). You can experiment when running to see what angle works better for you.

---

[19] Obviously you don't have to be a Bagua master to have an intuitive understanding of the *baihui*. People throughout the world have been using their heads in efficient ways for aeons. As with maintaining balance, discovering your *baihui* requires constant searching. You are searching for the feeling of pushing up from the top of your head in a way that makes you feel tall, strong, at ease, and confident all at the same time. The taller, stronger, and more at ease you feel, the more you know that your *baihui* is rising toward the sky.

Lesson 15
Reaching Up[20]

This lesson involves the supremely rejuvenating activity of skipping, and it provides a nice complement to both Lesson 9, "Reaching Up While Throwing," and Lesson 13, "Behind Your Behind." One reason I enjoy skipping is because it allows me to feel very light, as if I'm floating. In fact, for a split second during the skipping action, I *am* floating—and I imagine I'm Michael Jordan gliding through the air before dunking the ball. You can get enormous lift out of skipping—often more so than simply by jumping—such that participating in the activity might bring levity not just to your body but to your mood. Maybe a lack of skipping is one reason we adults and teenagers tend to be too serious. Skipping is such a delightful activity that it's a shame more of us don't do it. I myself stopped skipping for decades because it simply wasn't a "cool" thing to do once I became a teenager.

As with all other lessons, the constraints given in this one are intended to be used as tools for learning. They are not, therefore, rigid rules laid down for you to slavishly follow all the time and under all circumstances. For example, I include the constraint of dropping your tailbone and allowing your lower back to flatten and expand for you to discover new ways of configuring your spine, pelvis, and legs. This does not mean that it is normal to drop your tailbone and flatten your lower back *all the time.* No particular configuration for any part of your body is in fact appropriate for all circumstances. As I like to tell my students (and myself): "Use the constraint, but don't get used by it!" Starting Position: In standing, cross your arms at the wrists and interlace your fingers. Slowly bring your hands toward the sky. Your arms will come toward your ears and your elbows will begin to straighten.

1. Take your time to play with the gradual straightening of your elbows while bringing your arms backward as if you wanted to use them to squeeze the back of your head. Be gentle, as the goal is

---

[20] I first encountered elements of this lesson while studying Taichi in China and then years later while attending a training with Bones for Life founder and Feldenkrais Trainer Ruthy Alon.

not to "get there" but rather to go in the direction of straightening (without locking) the elbows.

A. Notice how your entire chest begins to lift. Also notice how your lower back begins to arch even more.

B. To counter the arching, drop your tailbone. You will feel your lower back flattening and the weight dropping more into your legs. Dropping your tailbone allows for an expansion of your lower back. Breathe down and back into this area and feel how it expands even more. Rest and walk around.

2. Resume the previous position, and this time, begin to walk. Lift your knees higher and higher, as if you were in the marching band. As you lift your knees, simultaneously straighten your elbows and reach for the sky with your hands. For most people, the resultant lifting of the rib cage will actually help to lift their knees higher.

A. Pause and allow your lower back to arch again before resuming marching. Notice the difference. Which do you prefer? Note that neither position is "right" nor "wrong." For people with a lordosis in the lumbar spine, dropping the tailbone can be

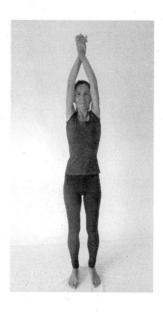 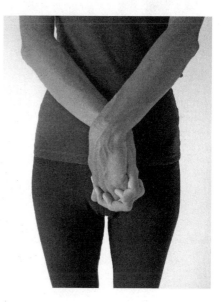

helpful in discovering new and possibly more efficient ways of standing, walking and running. Those of you with a lordosis may consequently find that this constraint gives you more propulsive power during the lesson. For the minority who use their spine in a healthy and efficient manner, dropping your tailbone during this lesson may or may not grant you more propulsive power—doing so may even hinder your power.

B. Experiment with arching your back more and even exaggerating the arch by sticking your tailbone up. Notice the difference in what you feel in your chest and in the relative ease or difficulty you have in lifting your knees.

C. Go back and forth with your tailbone—dropping it more, dropping it less, sticking it up more, or less, and see what the effect is on the positioning of your chest and on the lifting of your knees.

D. Rest.

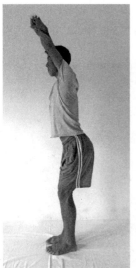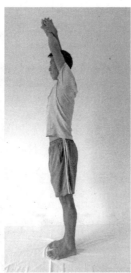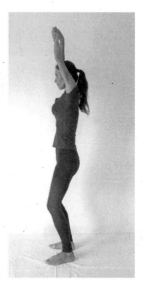

Pulling up the tailbone (left) versus dropping the tailbone (middle and right).

3. Resume the previous position of pulling up with the arms. Experiment with the dropping and lifting of your tailbone once again. Search for how to position your tailbone to give you more lift in your knees. Once you have found a more ideal position, begin to skip, lifting your knees higher and higher toward the sky. Each time you lift a knee, reach higher with your hands. Again, the lifting of your hands and thus your rib cage helps to pull your knees up. Feel how much lift and power you get as a result. Continue for a while, and whenever you want, drop your arms but continue skipping.

   A. Experiment with pumping each elbow backward and upward as it reaches behind you: as your left leg lifts, your left elbow pumps back and upward. See to it that you pump your arms as soon as you begin to rise upward. Be playful with each arm as it goes behind you. See what kind of motion gives you better lift.

   B. Experiment also with how you use each arm as it moves in front of your body. The motion of the arms should be quick and light.

   C. Rest and walk around when you feel like you've had enough.

4. Return to reaching for the sky with interlaced fingers (arms crossed). Begin walking, and at some point, begin skipping, using your arms to help lift your body.

   A. Whenever you want, drop your arms but continue skipping, noting the trajectory of your elbows.

   B. At some point, simply begin to run. See if you feel taller and more powerful. Does your stride feel easier? Rest whenever you want.

5. As an option, repeat any of the steps, but with your hands interlaced with the opposite hand in front.

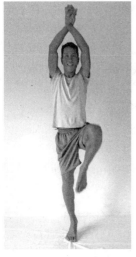 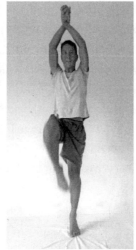 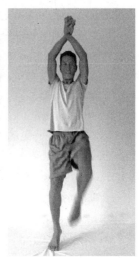

Marching.

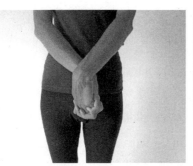 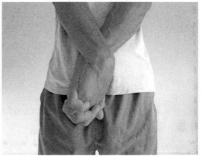

There are four principal variations for crossing and interlacing hands: with either wrist and either pinky on top; two possibilities are shown.

Lesson 16
Salsa Hips

Modern footwear, chairs, car seats, and even exercise and weight machines have contributed heavily to narrowing the ranges of motion in people throughout much of the Western world.[21] As mentioned earlier, popular

---

[21] For a fascinating history of how the chair has impacted human movement and form, see Galen Cranz, *The Chair: Rethinking Culture, Body, and Design* (*continued*)

footwear tends to act as a substitute for tendons, muscles, and your nervous system, thereby limiting what your body would otherwise do. The elevated and padded heels that we see in virtually all running shoes, for example, keeps your heels from reaching all the way to the earth and thereby prevents your spine from elongating (through rotation, side flexion, and extension) in order to facilitate that reach. The result is a weaker, less fluid, and less comfortable gait in walking and stride in running.

The following lesson will help to reinstate a suppleness in your pelvis and spine that is important for powerful walking and running. You may notice that in the ten to twenty minutes it takes to explore this lesson, the length of your gait has actually increased.

Starting Position: Stand with your feet about hip-width apart. Reach over the top of your head with your right hand such that the palm is somewhere on the crown and the fingers extend toward your left ear.

1. Begin to bring your right elbow down toward your right hip. Notice the first thing that moves. Repeat a few times, each time

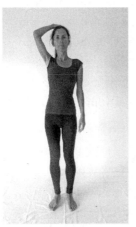 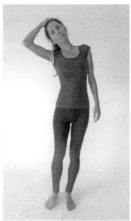 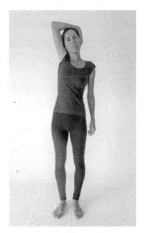

Left and middle: Make sure the bending is distributed evenly throughout your entire spine. Right: Note that you don't have to reach so far that your bicep touches your ear. If you reach that far, you could end up straining your neck.

(New York: W. W. Norton, 1998). For more on the limiting effect of exercise and weight machines, see Edward Yu, *The Mass Psychology of Fittism: Fitness, Evolution, and the First Two Laws of Thermodynamics* (Undocumented Worker Press, 2015).

with the intention of locating what moves first. This is likely the place from which you are initiating. Also notice how the weight shifts on your feet. Does it shift more to the right foot or to the left foot? It is important that you not stretch your neck during this lesson. In fact, I recommend minimizing the movement of your neck. How can you move your right elbow toward your right hip yet keep your neck from stretching at the same time?

2. Return to the starting position, and this time intentionally shift your weight to your left foot as your bring your right elbow toward your hip. Can you feel how much easier the movement becomes? Do this a few times and then compare it to shifting your weight onto your right foot while your elbow drops. Notice how shifting more to the right foot locks your pelvis and rib cage in place. To move farther, you have to stretch your upper body and your neck. Powerful movement generally relies on a more "democratic" distribution of work such that no one part gets stretched more than another. Continue once or twice and see to it that you are not stretching your neck in the process. Your neck should not feel any strain from these movements—if it does, stop immediately. Rest and notice how much longer you feel on one side compared to the other. Does your right arm feel longer? Is your right shoulder lower?

3. Return to the starting position and continue to explore the movement. This time notice that as you shift your weight to the left, your right heel gets lighter and lighter. Your right knee is bending. Allow your right hip to be totally free, and this will allow your leg to just "hang" from the joint. If you really allow it this freedom, you'll feel your right knee starting to point to the right even as it swings to the left. Go back and forth a few times, giving your right leg more and more freedom. Rest. The two sides of your body will feel more and more different.

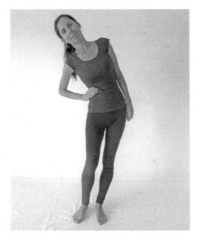

"Teapot" position.

4. Place your right hand on the right side of your rib cage with your thumb in back and the other four fingers in front. My students call this the "teapot" position (your right arm being the handle). Begin to lower your right elbow toward your right foot. Again, allow your weight to shift to your left foot. Feel how, like an accordion, the ribs on your right side squeeze together as your elbow goes down and come apart as your elbow comes up. This movement in the rib cage (called "side-bending") contains elements that are important to walking and running. Indeed, many movements in your rib cage are crucial to giving you power. Repeat a few times, then go back to the starting position with your hand on your head. Bring your elbow downward and see how much easier it is than when you started the lesson. Feel how your body is moving in unison. Rest.

5. Walk around and notice how much looser your right hip feels. Does your right foot reach farther forward with each step? Can you feel how your left shoulder is leading more than usual as you walk? Feel how you push off with more power in your left foot.

6. Repeat each step on the other side.

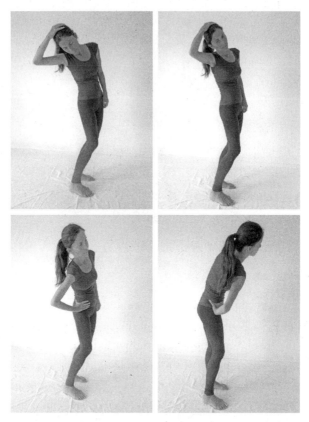

Avoid bending in any direction other than strictly sideways.
The examples above illustrate bending outside of the
desired plane.

Lesson 17
Reach and Roll on Your Back[22]

Starting Position: Lie on your back and bend your right leg so that your
right foot stands firmly on the floor.

---

[22] Note that step 6 of this lesson provides a nice complement to Lesson 24, "Rodin's Spiral,"
and Lesson 25, "Resistance as a Learning Tool," as well as step 3 of Lesson 6, "Screwing
Foot into Floor." For another take on some of the rotational aspects of this lesson, go to
Lesson 2, "Screwing Foot into Wall," and Lesson 27, "Where Does My Arm Begin?"

1. Begin to reach toward the ceiling with your right hand. Proceed a few inches, then reverse. Go back and forth, each time reaching a little farther toward the ceiling.

   A. What would prevent your arm from going farther, easily, and without a hint of discomfort? Ask yourself, "Where does my arm begin?"

   B. Notice if you've locked your elbow. If you have, bend it a tiny bit and continue.

   C. Don't go to a point of feeling strain or stretching anywhere in your neck, back, shoulder, or arm.

   D. Drop your arm and pause.

   E. With your arms down at your sides, gently push into the floor with your right foot. What happens to your right hip? What about your left hip? Push slowly, and release just as slowly.

   F. Go back and forth, each time pushing a little farther. Rest.

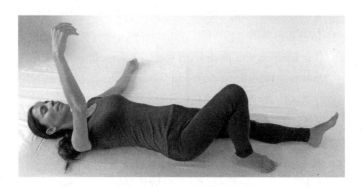

2. Resume pushing with your right foot (arms on the floor), but with the clear intention of rolling your pelvis a little to the left and then returning to neutral. Try it a few times and notice if the movement feels easier and completely different as a simple result of changing your intention. Could it be that following the instruction "Push into the floor" led you to unconsciously lift your entire pelvis—the heaviest part of your body—off the floor? Doing so would indeed

require a lot of effort. Yet, the greatest shifts in power usually occur through finding the easiest way to perform an action.

A. Continue looking for an easier, less effortful way to move. Is your left knee locked? See if you can let go of your left leg (unlock the knee if it is locked), thereby allowing your leg to roll to the left.

B. When you allow your pelvis to roll, your back turns to the left, beginning at the base of the lower back and traveling upward in a spiral—possibly all the way up to your neck. Continue slowly rolling your pelvis to the left and returning to neutral, each time sensing how your spine moves. Rest.

3. Return to the same configuration, and this time experiment with placing your right foot in different locations. Each time you push from a new location, feel how different the movement is in your knee, hip, and back. A simple shift of one inch in any direction will significantly alter the way your body moves. Try at least five different locations, pausing to rest whenever you want to. Pause.

A. Knowing you are going to roll your pelvis to the left, place your right foot where you feel you will have the most power.

B. This time, as you push with your foot, reach for the ceiling with your right hand. Though your body will roll to the left, your hand can continue reaching toward the ceiling. What are you doing with your head?

C. Go back and forth a few times, rolling to the left while reaching toward the ceiling. Keep the movement gentle and slow, noticing which is moving faster, your right shoulder or your right hip.

D. Rest with your arms at your sides and your legs long.

4. Prepare to reach and roll, but this time, reach over your right shoulder with your left hand so that you can hold it. As you reach for the ceiling with your right hand, use your left hand to pull on your right shoulder blade, thereby helping to roll your body to the left.

You will feel your left elbow turning to the left as you pull. Continue pushing with your right foot.

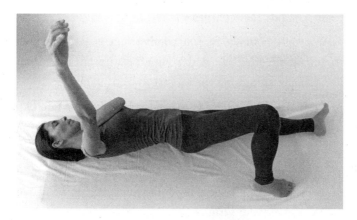

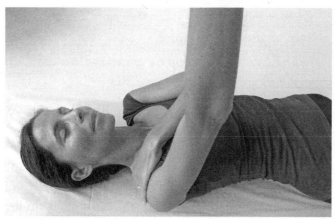

A. With each iteration, see if you can move more in synchrony—the right hand, left elbow, and right hip moving all at the same time.

B. Notice if your head wants to roll, and if so, in which direction?

C. Repeat a few times, then rest.

5. Repeat the previous step, but this time make a loose fist with your right hand and imagine that your first two knuckles form the blade of a screwdriver. As your right arm reaches toward the ceiling, begin to rotate the screwdriver.

   A. Your fist should be turning counterclockwise. (If you are exploring on the other side with your left fist toward the ceiling, then it should be turning clockwise.)

   B. Notice if the rotation helps your body roll to the left. Do you feel your head rolling to the left? If you don't, intentionally roll your head as you reach for the ceiling.

   C. Spiraling your arm this way may in fact release tension in your neck and shoulders and make the rolling easier. Ask yourself, "Where does my arm begin?"

   D. Go back and forth a few times, then place your arms on the floor.

   E. Push once or twice slowly with your right foot and notice how much easier the movement has gotten and how much looser your back and neck have become. Rest.

6. Advanced Step 1: Repeat the previous step, but this time reach *under* your armpit with your left hand. See if you can get a decent hold of your rib cage with this hand. If you are very flexible you'll be able to touch the bottom corner of your shoulder blade. Pulling in this manner, with your hand *under* the shoulder blade, will act to mobilize your spine to move differently than it did in the previous steps when you were reaching *over* it.

   A. Make a loose fist with your right hand. This time as you lift your hip and reach for the ceiling, turn the screwdriver in the opposite direction—that is, clockwise. (If you are exploring on the other side, with the left hand reaching toward the ceiling, the left hand should turn counterclockwise.)

   B. Allow your arm to bend as it spirals toward the ceiling.

   C. Go back and forth gently.

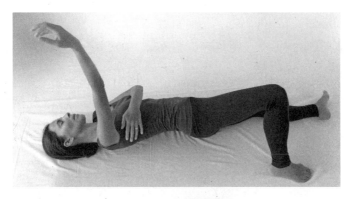

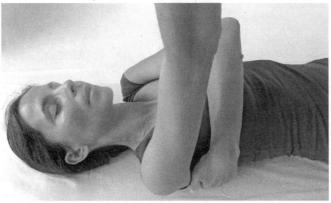

Rotating the hand in the opposite direction: hold under your shoulder blade with the opposite hand.

D. What does your head want to do?

E. Normally, configuring your body this way will bring your right shoulder a little closer to your right foot as you roll, thereby allowing the chest to expand. (Or another way to think of it: as your chest expands, it will prompt your shoulder to move toward your foot.) Your head may slide and tilt upward as if you wanted to look up and see what is resting on the floor just above your head. It may also want to roll, but in a different manner than during step 5. Whatever you do, make sure your

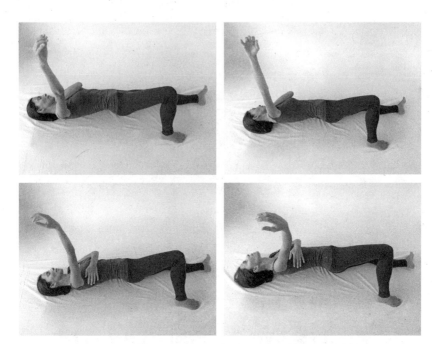

Spiraling the hand internally-medially (above) leads the spine differently than does spiraling it externally-laterally (below). Notice how Andreia's head, neck, and back respond differently, depending on which way her hand is spiraling.

> neck is comfortable! (If you are confused about what your head could or should be doing, don't try harder or make the movement larger and more forceful. Instead, make the movements *much smaller* and *slower* and sense how your neck responds. If you are still confused after trying this, take a rest and come back to this part later, or save it for another day—your neck will thank you for your patience!)

F. As you go back and forth, see to it that your jaw is loose. Notice if you are holding your breath at any moment.

G. Rest after a few iterations.

7. Advanced Step 2: Go back to the previous configuration, but this time place the knuckles of your right hand against the right side of your jaw. (Your right arm can be resting on top of your left wrist or

forearm.) You will look like a reclining version of Rodin's *Thinker*.
Begin to pull with your left hand and extend your right hip.

A. Notice if there is any tension or discomfort in your neck. (If
there is, stop immediately and rest.)

B. Go back and forth a few times, sensing how different everything feels when your hand is against your jaw.

C. Where does your right elbow want to go as you roll? Try
increasing the trajectory of your right elbow half an inch and
see how that affects the movement.

D. Rest whenever you want, then get up and walk around, noticing
the significant change on one side of your body.

8. When you are ready, lie down and go through each step on the
other side.

Lessons 18–19
"Boxer's Shuffle" Series

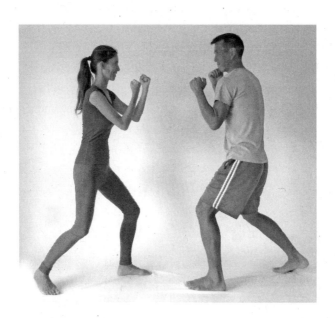

The following two lessons are the only ones in the book that are focused on improving both your strength and conditioning as well as your awareness. The reason for this is that most runners I have encountered, including those who lift weights and can leg press a good amount of weight, actually have functionally weak feet and legs. This could be explained by the fact that functional strength—the kind employed in the real world—is qualitatively different from the kind necessary to move the levers and pulleys attached to weight machines.

Since strength and conditioning are an important part of this series, I suggest you start slowly as always, but unlike with the other lessons, gradually increase your workload over the course of days, weeks, or months. In other words, push yourself from time to time. For even though all work and no play will indeed make Jack a dull boy and Jane a dull girl, all play and no work will likely turn both into pile of Jell-O. That said, please don't interpret this as an invitation to torture yourself. Rather, I hope you see it as an opportunity to challenge your physical stamina from time to time and to do so at a sensible pace.

Keep in mind that while challenging yourself, it is easy to lose sight of the given constraints, and in the process allow your form to crumble. To counter this tendency, I recommend you check yourself in the mirror now and again while playing with the movements in this series. If you want to go one step farther, videotape yourself.

As a final note, look for improvement rather than perfection. These lessons can be quite challenging in the beginning, but they will get easier over time. With regular practice, your legs and feet will become significantly stronger, and you may even begin to feel more agile.

Lesson 18
Getting Down

PART 1: FIRST APPROXIMATION

Starting Position: Standing.

1. Begin by standing with your feet hip-width apart, then stepping forward and throwing the ball just as you did in Lesson 1, "Posing

Questions." Throw easily without a great amount of force and freeze at the end of each throw, checking for balance and the positioning of different parts of your body.

A. Continue throwing, freezing, and adjusting, seeking positions that offer you more balance.

B. Once you have found a more optimal position at the end of your throw, drop your arm, observe the placement of your feet, and proceed to the next step.

C. At this point you can place your hands in various positions: at your sides, behind your back, or balled into loose fists, and placed near your chin.

2. Take a small step forward with your front foot—limiting the step to just a few inches—and then follow with your back foot. Maintain the distance between the two feet. This means your back foot will travel the same distance as your front foot. Continue for five steps with each foot. Then take a small step backward with your back foot and follow with your front foot. Continue for five steps.

A. When stepping forward, step first with your front foot. When stepping backward, step first with your back foot.

B. Go back and forth, limiting each step to only a few inches. Make sure you pick up either foot when you step, rather than sliding it. Also make sure your back heel stays off the floor.

C. Start to speed up your shuffling. Keep the steps small, but make them quick.

D. Rest after a few rounds of back and forth.

3. Resume shuffling and this time freeze during transition from going forward to backward. Are you leaning forward? (Many people cannot tell at first, so this is where a mirror might come in handy.) Slow down even more if it helps prevent you from leaning. Attention to detail during this transition is important in teaching you

how to stabilize your trunk and keep your upper body directly over your pelvis.

   A. Continue shuffling and freeze during the transition from backward to forward. Are you leaning backward? Again, minimize any leaning. Slow down for a while before gradually speeding up if doing so allows you to stay within the given constraints of the lesson.

   B. Go back and forth a few times before resting.

   C. Walk and notice the difference. Your right foot will feel very different from your left. Even your arms and shoulders may feel different from each other.

4. Repeat all the steps on the other side.

PART 2: "BOXER'S STANCE"

Starting Position: Return to your basic shuffling stance.

1. This time slowly drop your tailbone such that your lower back begins to flatten.

   A. As your tailbone drops, allow the center of your chest to cave inward. You should feel yourself getting shorter. If you continue the trajectory of your tailbone and chest, your tailbone will begin to curl forward and your chest will cave in even farther.

   B. Continue rounding until you reach your comfortable limit and pause for a moment. In this configuration your back should be rounded like a turtle shell, and you will feel significantly shorter.

   C. Slowly reverse the movement. In reverse, the center of your chest will eventually begin to push forward and upward. You should feel your chest rising and expanding while your tailbone begins to rise, curling in the opposite direction. The natural curve in your lower back will return. Begin to exaggerate the movement such that your tailbone starts to rise toward the ceiling as your chest thrusts forward and up. In this position your

. back will be strongly curved in the opposite direction from the previous step.

D. Go back and forth, noticing when your tailbone starts moving faster than your chest or vice versa. Begin synchronizing the movement so that your chest and tailbone move more in unison.

E. Rest.

2. Resume flexing and extending your back, once again exaggerating the movement at the very end: at one extreme your spine will go into a fetal-like position with your head down; in the other, your chest and belly will be wide open with your rear end sticking out and your nose pointing well above the horizon.

A. Notice that when the back is convex like a turtle shell, your legs have to work more.

B. Go back and forth a few times before resting.

3. Repeat the previous movement, but gradually make the movement smaller and smaller. Search for the point at which your lower back feels flat—neither convex nor concave. In this configuration you may feel a little slouched—at least compared to when you are standing tall. At the same time you will feel your legs really waking up.

A. Go back and forth, each time making the movement smaller. Your entire spine should be responding even though the movement is getting smaller.

B. When you think you've discovered the place where your lower back is flat, hold that position. For the sake of convenience, I'll call this the "boxer's stance" (even though it's missing some constraints to make it a true boxer's stance).

C. Now begin to shuffle forward, front foot stepping forward first. Keep the steps small and make sure not to slide your feet. As usual, keep your back heel off the floor. Go five steps and then reverse, back foot stepping first. Notice that maintaining the boxer's stance results in your legs and feet having to work much more than before.

D. Go back and forth slowly enough that you can start noticing when the configuration of your back begins to stray from where you want it.

E. When you feel more stable, you can begin to increase the speed of your shuffling. Make sure the front foot does not step farther than the back foot, or vice versa. Pause frequently to check the configuration of your chest and tailbone. With time, practice, and improved awareness, it will become easier to maintain a flat back.

F. Rest and walk around whenever you want to.

4. Repeat all the steps from part 2 on the other side. Then walk around and notice if your chest feels like it's floating.

PART 3: SHUFFLING SIDEWAYS

Starting Position: Return to the "boxer's stance."

1. Notice where the front of your back foot and the back of your front foot are on the floor. Tape two pieces of masking tape in two parallel lines on the floor in order to demarcate the desired distance between your feet. The lines should be roughly seven feet long.

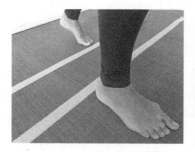 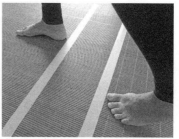

A. Place your front foot in front of the front line and the back foot behind the back line. Take a step to the left: step first with your left foot and then your right. Keep your steps small and make sure you lift your feet rather than sliding them.

B. Continue for five steps, then reverse and begin stepping to the right. When going to the right, step first with your right foot.

C. Go back and forth, taking five steps in each direction and making sure that you don't cross the line with either foot. (By doing so, you will be maintaining the original distance between your feet.) Pause frequently to check your stance.

D. Gradually increase the speed of your stepping. Notice if your head starts to bob up and down when the steps get faster. In other words, notice if you become a little taller in the middle of each step.

E. Rest whenever you want to.

F. As you repeat this lesson with some regularity, you will find that you can go faster and continue for longer periods without tiring.

2. Repeat all the steps from part 3 on the other side. When you are finished, walk and notice the difference in your feet, legs, and back. Do your feet roll off the floor with more clarity and power? Does your gait feel more fluid? You may be surprised that upon emerging from a low stance with a flat back, your chest feels lighter and more open and your neck longer.

Lesson 19
Staying Level-Headed

Starting Position: Return to the "boxer's stance" from the previous lesson. This time, have a partner stand in front of you, holding a yardstick, foam tube, or some other long object so that one end barely touches the top of your head. Have your partner keep both ends of the stick at the same height so that it is parallel to the floor. This is the height below which you want to stay for most of this lesson.

1. Begin shuffling forward (front foot first) with your partner keeping the yardstick at the desired height. As you shuffle, keep your head underneath the yardstick; this will prevent you from bobbing up and down.

A. In order to stay below the yardstick, you may have a tendency reach your chin forward and up the way people often do when they are sitting in the first row of a movie theater. You may also find yourself leaning forward from your waist. Neither action conforms to the given constraints. If your neck or back starts to feel bad, it's an indication that something is off. I recommend you stop frequently to check your positioning so as to avoid ending up with a neck- or backache.

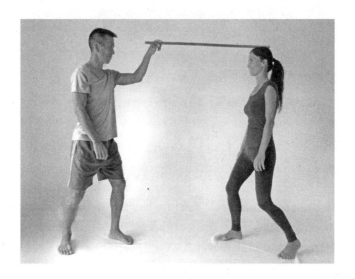

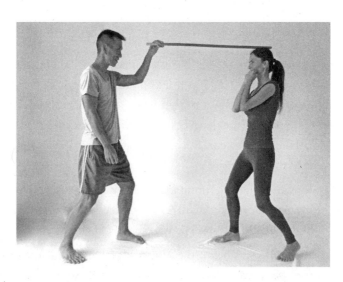

    B. After five steps, stop and shuffle backward (back foot first).

    C. Go back and forth slowly.

    D. Rest after a few trials.

2. Resume shuffling forward and backward slowly. Gradually increase your speed.

    A. When does your ability to abide by the constraints begin to break down? For example, is there a point at which you start to bob up and down? When do you start to arch your lower back or neck? When do you start to lean?

    B. Slow down or stop whenever you feel that you are losing control.

    C. Rest whenever you want.

3. Resume the boxer's stance, but this time, have your partner stand at your left side while holding the yardstick at the appropriate height. Begin stepping to the left (left foot first).

    A. Make sure you maintain the proper distance between your feet. (That would be the distance you established in previous lesson. If it helps you to maintain this distance, tape two parallel lines on the floor to mark it off before you begin stepping.)

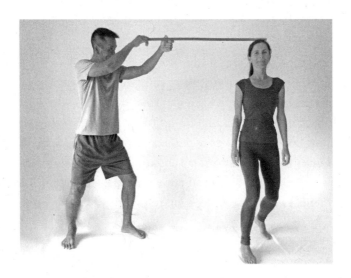

B. Shuffle slowly left and right, going five steps in each direction. Notice which direction is easier.

C. Rest after a few rounds.

4. Resume shuffling left and right, slowly increasing your speed.

A. Slow down frequently to check your positioning.

B. Rest after a few rounds.

5. Walk and notice if your chest feels lighter and your shoulders lower. Feel how clearly your feet roll off the floor.

Lesson 20

Making Your Head Lighter [23]

Starting Position: Lie on your back and feel how your shoulders are resting on the floor. Notice how wide they feel. Do they make much contact with the floor? Also notice how high the arch in your lower back is. Is it higher or lower than the arch in the back of your neck? Is your neck uncomfortable? If so, fold some towels neatly and place them under your head until your neck no longer feels strained. Slowly lift your head an inch off the floor to feel how heavy it is, then let it rest back on the floor. Take an estimate from 1 to 10, where 10 means your head is very heavy like a boulder, and 1 means it's very light and easy to lift.

1. Bend your knees so that your feet are flat on the floor and about hip-width apart. Start to press gently with your feet. Do you feel your pelvis moving? What about your lower back? Press gently and let go gently. Go back and forth slowly, noticing if your pelvis is tilting and if your lower back is coming toward the floor. When the muscles in the lower back are chronically tense, they will hold the spine like an iron board and prevent it from curving easily into the ground. Lengthen your legs and rest.

---

[23] Lesson 14, "Water Jugs, Furniture, and Other Things to Carry on Your Head," provides a different perspective on some of the motor concepts developed in this lesson.

2. Imagine that your spine is a keyboard. With the fingers of either hand, press into three "keys" in your lower spine (if for some reason you cannot reach your lower back with your hand, have somebody else do it for you). Once you have a clear sense of those three keys, remove your hand.

   A. Push with your feet, and one by one, begin to bring each of the three keys you just located toward the floor. If your lower back is tense, you may need to engage your abdominal muscles in order to do this. Note that it isn't imperative that the three keys actually touch the floor. They only need to go toward the floor.

   B. Once you have done this, slowly reverse the movement so that the keys move away from the floor one by one. Go back and forth slowly, clearly feeling each point either touching or coming toward the floor. See if you can do the movement more and more smoothly. Notice if you are veering off to the right or left. Go slowly enough so that you can notice how precisely you are traveling up the middle of your spine.

   C. Continue decreasing your speed until it takes five seconds to get all three points on the floor, and five seconds to reverse the movement. You may want to count slowly to yourself, "One … two … three …" in order to make sure you are really slowing down.

   D. Rest with your legs long.

3. Bend your knees again, and this time, begin to raise your lower back from the floor, making the arch higher. You can do this by rolling your pelvis forward and letting go of, or even pushing out, your lower abdomen. Rather than sucking in your gut, you will be letting it hang out as the arch in your back rises. Go back and forth a few times before resting.

4. Feel the back of your head resting on the floor. Imagine you have some paint on that part of your head and you want to wipe it off onto the floor by sliding your head up and down, as if to nod.

   A. Your chin will move toward your chest and away from your chest as you do this. Remember that you are sliding your head, not lifting it—your head should stay in contact with the floor in order to wipe the paint off. See to it that you make the movement smooth and easy. This is not intended to be a workout for your neck, and it is not intended to stretch the neck, so be very gentle. The movements do not have to be large.

B. What is it that prevents your head from moving farther and more easily? Can you feel any movement in the center of your chest? What could your chest be doing in order to make the movement easier? Go back and forth several times.

C. Rest.

5. Touch the bottom of your breastbone. To either side of this point you will discover a set of ribs branching off. Place the heels of your hands on these ribs—the left hand will press on the left branch, the right hand on the right branch. Have your fingers pointing in the direction of your pelvis.

A. Raise your elbows a little and start to press with the heels of your hands as if you wanted to tuck your ribs downward into your pelvis. (Another way to think of this is to imagine that your upper body forms a big ball of dough with an air pocket beneath it. The air pocket is the arch in your lower back. By pressing with the heels of your hands, you are flattening the dough and squeezing out the air pocket. The motion is similar to the motion of kneading bread.)

B. Allow your lower back to come toward the floor as you press—this is what will allow the ribs to move. See to it that you press with the heels of your hands and not with your fingers. This will give you more power. Go back and forth several times slowly, trying to feel how the lower back can sink toward the floor. Can you feel your chest moving? Pause.

C. Begin to slide your head on the floor as you push your ribs down toward your pelvis. Your chin moves away from your chest as you push (the back of your head slides toward the area between your shoulder blades), and moves back toward your chest as you stop pushing.

D. Rest with your arms and legs long.

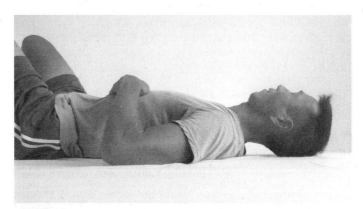

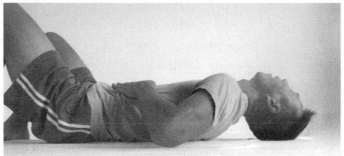

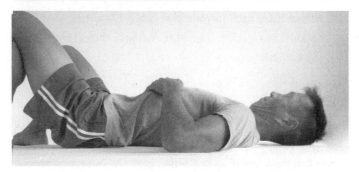

These photos show fairly large movements of the neck, chest, and lower back. I recommend you start with tiny movements until you can feel your lower back responding to even the slightest up-down sliding of your head.

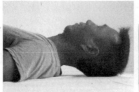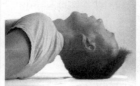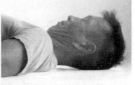

Note how much my shoulders and chest respond to the sliding of my head.

6. Bend your legs and stand with your feet on the ground about hip-width apart. Press gently into the floor with both feet. Notice if your lower back sinks more easily to the floor now. Can you feel those three points more distinctly touching the floor as you press? Go back and forth a few times very slowly and notice if your chest moves as you push. Notice if your head moves as well. If you sense more movement in your chest and head, it means that chronically tense muscles between your hips and your chest and head have let go. Excessive muscle tension, in other words, is no longer blocking the force from traveling all the way up your spine.

   A. Place your hands on your ribs and simply slide your head on the floor as you did earlier. Go slowly. Can you feel your ribs moving and lower back sinking? Even without pressing with your hands, your ribs may move automatically. Rest with arms and legs long.

   B. Notice if the arch in your lower back has gotten lower. Does the back of your neck feel longer? Are your shoulders resting more comfortably into the floor?

7. Take your time to roll over and sit up and eventually stand up. Once in standing, close your eyes and notice how low and relaxed your shoulders are. They may feel like they are just hanging off your body, no longer rising with tension. Do you feel taller? Does your chest feel more open, as if it is floating? Do you feel more rooted in your feet? Walk around slowly and feel how comfortable walking is. The exploration on the floor has changed your muscle tone and woken up connections that have long been dormant.

Lessons 21–26
"Metatarsals to Metacarpals" Series

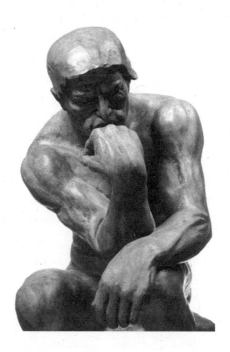

Inspired in part by a set of advanced Feldenkrais lessons that I encountered during my training to become a Feldenkrais Practitioner, the "Metatarsals to Metatarsals" series asks for a good deal of flexibility in the feet (including dorsiflexion in the toes), knees (flexion), hips (extension), lumbar spine (extension), and thorax (extension).[24] As with any series of movements that demand greater ranges of motion, this series of lessons will put you at greater risk for injury if you do not proceed incrementally and respect your

---

[24] The advanced lessons I am referring to are part of what Feldenkrais Practitioners call the "Sitting on the Heels" series. I call them "advanced" because they were too difficult for me to complete during my training, despite the fact that I was relatively young (in my early thirties) at the time, and had been athletic my entire life.

limits. For those of you lacking flexibility in your feet, knees, or back (that would be most adolescents and adults in the West, and a growing number of their cohort in other parts of the world), proceed extremely slowly. In fact, start by exploring only the tiniest of movements and resting frequently. Consider spreading the entirety of any given lesson over the course of several days, weeks, or even months—perhaps exploring just one small portion of it at a time. If, during any part of any lesson, you experience intense stretching in any of your toes, the soles of your feet, quadriceps, or lower back, then you are probably going way too far for your own good. Keep in mind that by proceeding too quickly or forcefully, you may end up on the surgeon's table.[25] If you have had any prior injuries to your knees or feet, you might even consider skipping this series altogether. Also keep in mind that the primary goal of these lessons is not to increase your flexibility. Rather, it is for you to improve your sense-ability and awareness and thereby discover how seemingly disparate parts of your body can work together in a cooperative manner.

Lesson 21
Walking While Sitting

Exploring one or more of the "Metatarsals to Metacarpals" lessons can over time help to make up for the decreases in strength, flexibility, balance, and agility that normally result from becoming dependent on chairs. If, like me, you grew up sitting on chairs, you will likely find this lesson to be quite challenging. If, on the other hand, you spent much of your life on the floor, like people in most of the non-Western world, this lesson will be a piece of cake. Either way, it is important to go slowly so that you can discover how it is you actually move, what your habitual preferences are, and where your subsequent biases lie. Being able to perform a movement quickly doesn't necessarily mean you perform it well, or even that you have much awareness of how you are performing it.

---

[25] This is one reason I generally do not recommend anything beyond mild stretching during any lesson or even as a preparation for exercise.

Starting Position: Sit on the floor with your legs in front, knees slightly bent and out to the sides. How comfortable is your back? Can you sit without propping yourself up with your hands?

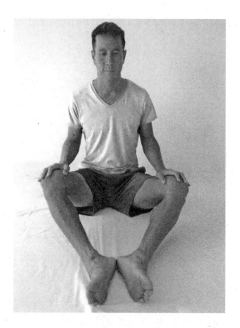

1. Lift your right knee until the sole of the right foot is facing the floor. Make sure your hands are not touching the floor. What happens with your trunk when you lift your right knee? Does your right buttock lift off the floor?

   A. Let your knee slowly drop back down to the right, then bring it up again. Go back and forth a few times noticing where in your body you are making the effort and how your rib cage does or doesn't respond.

   B. Try a few times with your left knee and compare the difference. Which side is easier? Pause and rest for a few moments. (In resting you can put your hands on the floor if you want.)

C. Lift your right knee again. If it isn't already lifting, make sure that your right buttock also lifts. You will feel muscles on your right side engaging. You may feel your shoulder swinging in one direction or another. Go back and forth, slowly lifting and then gradually dropping your right buttock.

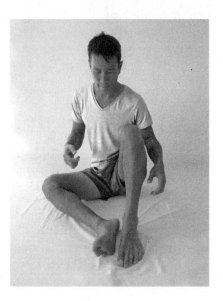

D. Switch sides and notice if the left buttock is easier or more challenging to lift than the right. Slowly go back and forth between lifting the right and the left.

E. Rest on your back.

2. Return to the starting position, and this time when you lift your right buttock, bring it forward and let it drop onto the floor again. Then lift it and move it back to its original position.

A. Go back and forth a few times, feeling how your trunk and shoulders respond.

B. Switch sides and compare which buttock is easier to move back and forth. Pause and rest.

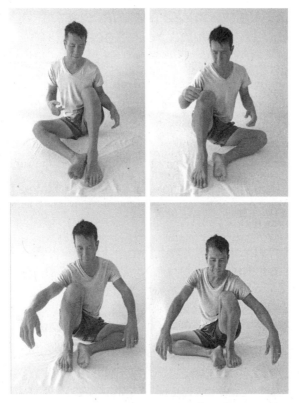

From upper left clockwise to lower left: walking on the sit bones toward the feet.

3. Begin to walk your buttocks forward toward your feet (leaving your feet where they are). How close can you bring your buttocks to your feet? Which buttock gets closer—right buttock to right foot, or left buttock to left foot?

   A. Once you are as close as you can get to your feet, begin to walk your buttocks backward, moving away from your feet. Play with walking your buttocks toward your feet and away.

   B. When you are ready, stand up and walk around, sensing the differences in your posture and in your gait. Notice if the sides of your trunk feel more alive.

Lesson 22 (Advanced)[26]
Driving Your Knees

(Make sure you have completed the previous lesson before starting this one.)

Finding a stronger connection between the dorsiflexion of your feet, acute flexion of your knees, and extension of your hips and thorax is important not only for providing greater health and comfort to your feet, knees, hips, and entire spine (from your sacrum to the base of your skull), but for generating increased propulsive power in both walking and running.

Starting Position: Sit on the floor with your legs in front, knees slightly bent and out to the sides (the same as in the previous lesson). Don't let your hands touch the floor.

1. As in the previous lesson, walk your buttocks toward your feet. Once you have walked your buttocks as close to your feet as they can reach, place your fists with palms facing inward, on the floor near your buttocks. As an option, you can instead place your palms flat on the floor, place each palm on a bolster or brick, or place your hands in a tripod position (see the image below). The more flexible you are and the stronger your shoulders and abdominal region, the lower your wrists can be. Conversely, the less flexible you are and the less conditioned your shoulders and abdominal region, the higher your wrists will need to be. (The lowest position for your wrists would be to have your palms flat on the floor.)

---

[26] Perhaps even more than with other lessons, advanced lessons should be approached with great care and attention, since any given step may make demands on parts of your body that have been dormant for a long time. To reduce your risk of injury: (1) be prepared to stop frequently and spread the lesson over days, weeks, or even months; (2) avoid any movements that result in a feeling of intense stretching. If you feel intense stretching in any part of yourself, you are probably going *way* too far; (3) consider skipping any part that feels risky.

A. With your feet flat on the floor, lift your pelvis and your heels. You'll notice that the lifting involves not only your calf muscles but your shoulders, back, and abdominal region.

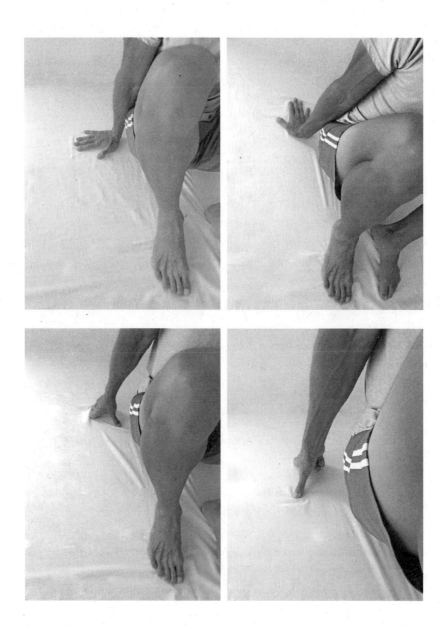

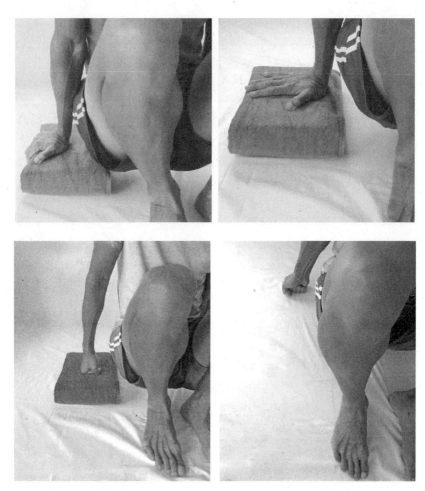

Some different possibilities for hand placement, both with and without a brick.
There are obviously possibilities not shown here, so don't be afraid to experiment.

B. See if you can lift the heels high with only your toes and the balls of feet touching the floor. For many this will be a challenging movement because it involves lifting the entire pelvis and trunk toward the ceiling. Are you holding your breath when you lift your heels? If you find that you cannot lift your heels off the floor without holding your breath, stop and return to this lesson on another day.

C. Go back and forth, lifting your pelvis and heels and bringing them back down. Notice if you start to constrict your breathing whenever you begin to lift your heels.

D. Rest on your back.

2. Repeat step 1, but this time, once your heels are lifted, keep them lifted and slowly bring your pelvis over your heels. Continue gently pushing your pelvis forward so that your knees will begin to tilt downward toward the floor in front of you. Take note if, upon reading the last line, you had a sudden urge to bring your knees *to* the floor and not simply *toward* the floor.

A. Proceed incrementally. Tilt just a little, perhaps only a few inches, then return. Each time, go a little farther, as long as it is not a strain to do so.

B. You will feel your toes stretching. You will also feel your chest and shoulders opening up. Go only as far as is comfortable for your feet, chest, and shoulders. Avoid any forceful, painful, or otherwise intense stretching.

C. Notice which toes in your left foot begin to stretch. Notice how differently it feels in your left foot compared to your right. Notice also how differently it feels in your left hip compared to your right, and your left shoulder compared to your right.

D. Experiment with putting the knees either farther apart or closer together as you tilt them downward.

E. If and when at some point you are able to bring your knees to touch the floor without straining, experiment with looking up and behind you, as if you wanted to scan the wall behind you. Notice how the farther away your chin comes from your chest, the more your chest opens up and the less pulling you feel in the front of your thighs.

F. Rest on your back.

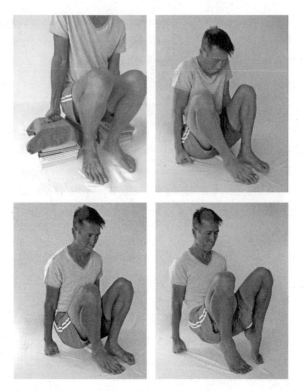

Step 1. Note the option of sitting on a stool or a bolster
(top left).

3. Return to having your buttocks close to your heels, and your hands
   on the floor with palms facing inward. (If your palms are resting
   flat on the floor or on bolsters, keep your fingers pointing either
   backward or out to the sides.)[27] Resume where you left off in
   step 2: tilt your knees toward the floor.

   A. Go back and forth, incrementally increasing the tilting of your
      knees. If your knees were to continue in their trajectory, where
      would they eventually touch the floor?

   ───────────

   [27] Having your fingers pointing forward during the following explorations will limit your
   range of motion and put the unnecessary stress on your shoulders. Thus, to increase
   your range of motion and simultaneously protect your shoulders, keep your fingers
   pointing either outward or backward.

B. Pause with your knees tilting comfortably toward the floor. In this position, lead with your right knee, bringing your right knee *toward* the midline. In other words, instead of bringing your knee downward in its original trajectory, direct it slightly inward so that it goes toward the midline. At the same time, allow your left knee to splay outward and farther to the left. Notice how your trunk bends sideways and the right side of your chest opens up. Go back and forth a few times, noticing the effect on your chest and right shoulder.

C. Pause, and now lead with your left knee, bringing it toward the midline. Notice how different it is on this side. Go back and forth once or twice and then rest on your back.

4. Explore the previous step again, but this time pay attention to which knuckles carry more weight (or if your hands are resting on bolsters, which parts of your palm carry more weight). Make sure your palms are facing inward. (If your palms are resting flat on the floor or on bolsters, make sure your fingers point backward or outward to the sides.)

A. Experiment with having the weight on different knuckles (if you are balanced on your fists) or different parts of your palm (if you are balanced with palms down) and notice how this affects how far you can comfortably tilt your knees. How does changing the weight on your hands affect the feeling in your chest and shoulders? Pause after a few iterations.

B. Try rotating your forearms inward-medially (with your elbows turning outward) as your knees come toward the floor, and notice how this limits the movement. Go slow enough that you can notice the effects on your shoulders and chest.

C. Try rotating the forearms outward-laterally (with elbows turning inward) and notice how this increases your range.

D. Repeat a few times, then rest.

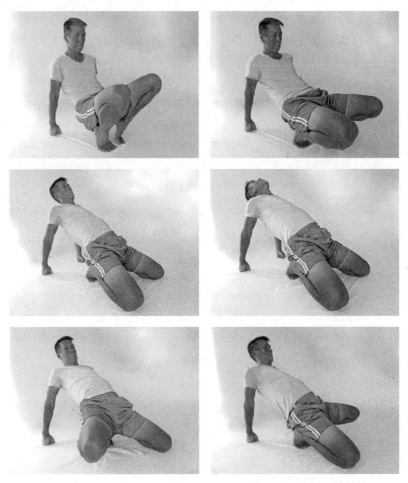

Middle right: If you are able to bring your knees to the floor easily, experiment with looking up in order to scan the wall behind you. Bottom left and right: bringing one knee downward and toward the midline.

5. Return to having your buttocks close to your heels and tilting your knees downward.

   A. Is it easier? Do you feel more movement in your rib cage and more mobility in your toes?

   B. Repeat a few times, checking to see what differences you feel from earlier in the lesson.

C. Over time—it may take weeks or months—you may find that you can touch the floor with either or both knees. Do not turn this into a rigid goal, but instead, view it as a possibility. If there is a goal, it is simply to observe how different parts of your body respond as you gently explore each movement.

D. Stand up and notice how rooted you feel in your feet and how light and open your chest feels. Walk around and see if you feel your feet rolling off the floor with greater clarity. Does your chest feel like it's floating? Do you feel taller?

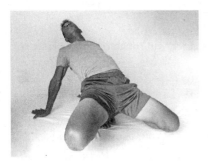 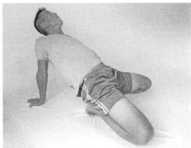

Look up and toward the wall behind you as either knee comes to the floor; your head will probably want to turn to one side or the other, depending on which knee comes to the floor.

Lesson 23 (Advanced)[28]
Driving Your Knees with a Twist (or Spiral)

(Make sure you have completed the previous two lessons before starting this one.)

---

[28] Perhaps even more than with other lessons, advanced lessons should be approached with great care, attention, and even a hint of caution since any given step could make demands on parts of your body that have been dormant for a long time. To reduce your risk of injury: (1) be prepared to stop frequently and spread the lesson over days, weeks, or even months; (2) avoid any movements that result in a feeling of intense stretching. If you feel intense stretching in any part of yourself, you are probably going *way* too far; (3) consider skipping any part that feels risky.

Starting Position: Sit on the floor with your legs in front and slightly bent, with the soles of your feet facing toward the middle (the same as in the previous two lessons). Don't let your hands touch the floor.

1. Begin to walk your buttocks toward your feet, just as you did in the previous two lessons. Once your buttocks are as close to your heels as you can comfortably bring them, straighten your left leg.

   A. Place your hands (in fists, tripods, or palms flat) on the floor next to your buttocks and lift your buttocks. Begin to push your right buttock over your right heel.

   B. Your left knee will automatically begin to bend and your right heel will begin to lift.

   C. At some point your right buttock will touch or come closer to touching your heel.

   D. Go back and forth, bringing your right buttock to your right heel, and then back to the floor.

   E. Much of the effort will come from your shoulders and back. Notice if you are digging your left heel into the floor, thereby engaging the hamstring muscles. Experiment with intentionally digging your left heel into the floor. Try digging with more effort and then try digging with less.[29] You may discover that the more you dig with your heel, the less effort you need from your shoulders and back.

   F. Rest momentarily in a comfortable sitting position.

2. Return to sitting with hands pushing the floor, your right buttock close to your right heel and your left leg straight in front of you.

---

[29] Note that some running experts describe the action of running as a pulling force whereby the hamstring and gluteal muscles pull the leg backward against the ground. Others refer to a pushing-off action whereby the calf muscles in coordination with the gluteal region push the body forward from the ball of the foot. Whether you want to think of pulling or pushing, it is vital to understand that both actions should involve the entire body, whereby the back, arms, and even neck work synergistically with the pelvis, legs, and feet.

Lift your pelvis and begin to bring your pelvis toward your right heel again.

A. This time go a little farther. Your pelvis will begin to roll over your right heel. Your left leg will bend more and more until your left foot is flat on the floor.

B. As your right knee moves forward, you will feel your chest opening up.

C. Rock back and forth on the ball of your right foot. Each time you rock forward, bring your right knee a little closer to the floor. Notice which toes are stretching. (If you feel intense stretching, then you are going way too far. You may want to skip the rest of the lesson and just explore the first two or three steps. Whatever you decide, I recommend you stay within your comfortable limits.)

D. Rest after a few iterations.

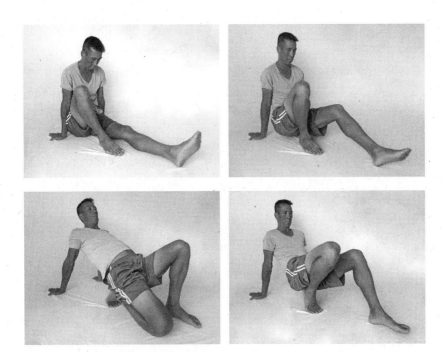

Clockwise from top left to lower left: steps 1 and 2.

3. Repeat the previous step, but this time point your right knee in different directions as it comes toward the floor. You'll notice that different toes will feel a stretch depending on the direction in which your knee points. You'll also feel differences in the way your chest opens and bends. Are you able to touch the floor comfortably with your knee? Are there directions for the knee to travel that are uncomfortable for your right foot, and particularly for certain toes?

   A. Continue exploring, noting which direction extends your big toe more, which direction extends your 2nd toe, and so on down to your 5th toe.

   B. Rest in sitting.

4. Repeat the previous step, and this time, focus on bringing your right knee straight down such that the pressure on the ball of your foot stays primarily between your big toe and 2nd toe.

   A. Notice how your left knee bends and automatically comes closer to the ceiling as your right hip extends and your right knee reaches closer to the floor. Conversely, as your right hip flexes and your right knee comes away from the floor, your left knee begins to straighten.

   B. Rest after a few iterations.

5. Return to rocking on the ball of your right foot, but this time, hold your right elbow against your rib cage such that your hand can rest on the left side of your chest and the fingers of your right hand can hold onto your left collarbone.

   A. Bring your right knee toward the floor again and notice how your trunk begins to turn to the left: the closer your knee gets to the floor, the more your trunk turns to the left.

   B. Go back and forth.

   C. What's happening in your left shoulder? In your left hand?

   D. Rest after a few iterations.

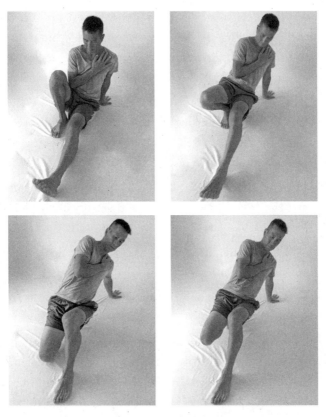

Clockwise from top left to lower left: does this movement
remind you of anything?

6. Repeat the previous step, and this time make sure your left hand is
in a fist with the palm facing to the right.

   A. Which knuckles of your left hand press down as you bring your
right knee to the floor?

   B. Experiment once or twice with pressing the last two knuckles
(those of the pinky and ring finger) into the floor. Then try
pressing down with the first two knuckles (those of the index
and middle fingers). Can you feel the difference in your left
shoulder? Chest? Hips?

   C. Rest.

7. Repeat the previous step, but this time bring the pressure on your left fist into the first two knuckles. As you bring your right knee toward the floor, begin to pronate your fist (rotate it clockwise). It's as if your first two knuckles form the blade of a screwdriver and you are attempting to drive a screw into the floor.

   A. The left fist will only move a tiny amount, if at all, because much of your body weight is resting on it. The entire left arm will begin to spiral in response.

   B. How does this spiraling of your hand affect your left shoulder and chest? How does it affect the trajectory of your left hip and left knee?

   C. When your right knee moves away from the floor, reverse the spiraling of your left fist.

   D. Go back and forth noticing how the spiraling affects your left hip and knee.

   E. By experimenting with different connections between the movement of the metacarpals (in the hands) and the metatarsals (in the feet), we can learn how the two can work synergistically with the spine, pelvis, and legs to increase propulsive force.[30]

   F. Rest.

---

[30] Tyson Gay, who is the former 100-meter world champion and the current U.S. record holder in the same event, understands this type of synergy well. Some believe that learning to spiral his hands in concert with the movement of the rest of his body helped him beat Usain Bolt in the Diamond League 100 meters back in 2010. According to one article: "Side views show Gay's forward hand rotating slightly outward at the wrist, his fingers curling slightly toward the base of the thumb. Exercise geeks call it supinating. His back arm is doing precisely the opposite, though to a lesser extent. It is pronating—rotating slightly inward at the wrist, with the palm facing the rear in a whipping action. His arms are basically making spiral movements.... He ran his best when he was spiraling the most. 'The one race I know for sure he used it was the Great City Games last May in Manchester [UK],' says Chase Kough, Gay's curly strength trainer. 'He said he focused on it the second half of the race.' In that race, Gay ran a 19.41, breaking a 44-year-old world record for a 200 race with no turns." Paul Scott, "The Revolutionary New Science of Speed," *Men's Health*, January 31, 2011.

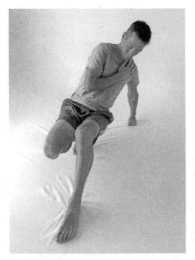
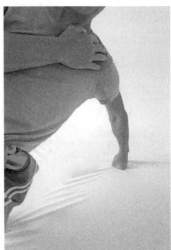

8. Repeat the previous step, but this time reverse the spiraling. In other words, as the right knee comes toward the floor, supinate your left fist (rotate it counterclockwise).

   A. Notice how different the movement becomes when you reverse the spiraling of the left fist. Notice how doing so increases the rotation of your trunk to the left.

   B. Play with this for a while before reversing the spiraling of the left fist once again such that it turns clockwise when your right knee comes toward the floor.

   C. Is it clearer now how the direction of spiraling affects the movement of the trunk and hips?

   D. When you are ready, rest on your back. Notice how different the two sides of your body feel. Which arm feels longer? Which leg? Which side of your trunk expands more when you breathe in?

9. Stand up and walk. See if you can feel that any one of the following connections has become clearer:

   Right hip to left knee

   Right foot to left knee

Left shoulder to left knee

Left shoulder to right foot

Left shoulder to right hip

Left hand to right foot

10. Stride easily around the room to see how different your right and left knees feel as they lift. Notice which shoulder is leading.

11. Repeat all the steps on the other side.

Lesson 24
Rodin's Spiral[31]

(Make sure you have completed the previous three lessons before starting this one.)

Starting Position: In standing, prepare to throw an imaginary ball with your right hand just as you did in Lesson 1, "Posing Questions."

PART 1: "THE THINKER"

1. Throw the ball a few times to get a sense of where you can place your feet and how you can stabilize your front leg in order to gain more balance and power.

   A. Continue adjusting your feet, searching for where you have more stability. Pay attention to the movement of your front knee. As you discovered in the "Throwing the Ball" series, your front knee should neither move forward nor inward (medially) while throwing if you want to maintain stability while increasing power.

   B. Drop your arm and simply rotate on your back foot. Aim to rest more of your weight on a different metatarsal each time you repeat the movement. Notice how ending closer to the 5th metatarsal

---

[31] Both Lessons 24 and 25 provide a nice complement to step 6 of Lesson 17, "Reach and Roll on Your Back," and step 3 of Lesson 6, "Screwing Foot into Floor."

changes not only how the back foot, ankle, and knee move, but also how the front knee spirals and how the front hip flexes.

C. Are you leaning forward? If so, adjust your upper body so that you are upright. In doing so, you will feel your right hip extending a little more.

D. Rest for a moment and notice how much bigger your right foot feels.

2. Repeat the previous step, but this time, as your right knee rotates leftward, allow it to simultaneously begin dropping toward the floor.

A. Most people will naturally stand up taller and bring their weight forward as they rotate. Dropping your knee toward the floor as you rotate prevents you from getting taller and keeps your center from moving forward. All of the force from your legs will consequently go strictly into rotating your pelvis and trunk. In this position, you will notice both your legs working more and the joints in your back foot stretching a little farther.

B. If you have a mirror handy, explore this movement while facing it and see if you can rotate without having your head tilt, turn, or otherwise move in any direction.

C. Go back and forth a few times, then rest.

3. Repeat the previous step and start to notice that changing where you rest on your back foot affects your front knee and front foot.

A. If you are very attentive, you will notice that your left knee spirals outward and backward (counterclockwise) during the movement. Notice that the spiral of your left knee will be tighter or wider depending on what you are doing with your right foot.

B. Begin to pay attention to your chest. How far does it rotate? How much does your upper back extend at the end of your rotation? If you had a laser shooting straight out of the center of your chest, where would it be pointing at the end of your rotation?

C. Rest after a few trials.

4. Repeat the previous step, but this time, end with your weight closer to the outside of your right foot—somewhere around the 4th or 5th metatarsal.[32] If you have a weak ankle that tends to get injured easily, stay close to the 1st and 2nd metatarsals. Make sure your back knee is dropping toward the floor as you rotate, thereby preventing you from getting taller at the end of the rotation.

A. You will notice that by allowing your weight to shift outward on your back foot, your ankle will bend a little more outward. You should feel stable here because it's roughly the same position the foot and ankle go into when you are on your tiptoes. (Again, if your ankle is vulnerable to injury, keep your weight closer to the 1st and 2nd metatarsals.)

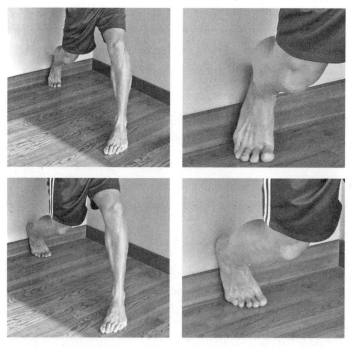

Weight distributed around the 1st and 2nd metatarsals (top) versus the 4th and 5th metatarsals (bottom).

---

[32] To get a better sense of the connection between the 4th and 5th metatarsals and extension and internal rotation of your hip, go to Lesson 6, "Screwing Foot into Floor."

B. Go back and forth a few times, noticing how ending on the outside of your foot automatically turns your trunk farther while opening up your chest.[33] Your trunk will be almost completely turned to the left.

C. Rest.

5. Repeat the previous step, but this time rest your right elbow against your rib cage and curl your right hand into a gentle fist, placing it under or against the right side of your jaw. Since you will look a little like Rodin's *The Thinker,* we'll call this position "The Thinker."

A. Go back and forth, keeping your head still. (Once again, this is easier to monitor if you are in front of a mirror.)

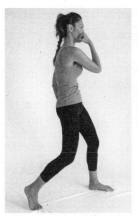
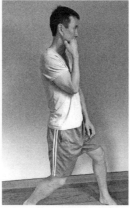
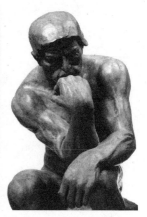

The right fist under or next to the chin. Left: There may be a tendency to stick your elbow far from your rib cage. Middle: the elbow attached to the rib cage. Right: Rodin's *The Thinker.*

---

[33] Compare this to previous lessons where rotating on the outer metatarsals while attempting to keep all other parts of the foot off the floor (including other metatarsals and all of your toes) prevented you from rotating farther in the medial direction. In contrast, keeping your weight to the outside of the ball of your foot while allowing the entire ball of the foot, along with the toes, to rest on the floor allows for a greater medial-internal rotation.

B. Notice how your entire body is actually rotating around your head. As long as you keep your head still and your arm glued to your rib cage, your fist will also be pivoting around your jaw.

C. Rest.

6. Repeat the previous step, and this time freeze at the end of your rotation. Straighten your left elbow so that your hand is somewhere behind your left buttock. Begin to rotate your left hand in one direction and then in the opposite direction.

   A. Rotating your left hand in one direction will bring the left shoulder backward and accentuate the rotation of your trunk. Rotating it in the opposite direction will bring the left shoulder forward and decrease the rotation of your trunk.

   B. Play with these movements as you discover how the rotation of your hand can affect the positioning of your shoulder and chest.

   C. Rest.

7. Rotate again, ending on the 4th and 5th metatarsals of your back foot. For now you can let your left arm drop, but keep your right hand on your chin. Begin to speed up at the very end of your rotation.

   A. Each time, go a little faster at the very end.

   B. Think of flicking your back heel outward.

   C. Pause.

8. Repeat the previous flicking motion, and this time allow your right elbow to slide forward at the very end of the movement so that it is no longer touching your rib cage. Imagine tapping a pad a few inches in front of your right elbow.

   A. The motion can be loose and easy as long as you allow the elbow to move at the end of the flicking motion.

   B. Notice how your right fist is pivoting or rotating around the right side of your jaw. Remember to keep your right fist loose.

   C. Move your imaginary pad a little to the right and continue. How does this affect the movement?

D. Move your imaginary pad to the left and continue. Notice how moving to your elbow farther across to the other side affects your spine, hip, and back foot. See if you can keep your head from moving.

E. Every now and then, freeze at the end of the motion and check your balance and the positioning of different parts of yourself.

F. Have fun with the movement. (Note that some of the body mechanics you are exploring here are also evident in the uppercut in boxing.)[34]

G. Rest whenever you want. When you are ready, walk around and feel the difference in your gait. One side may feel "new and improved" compared to the other.

9. Repeat all the steps on the opposite side (with your right leg forward). When you are finished, notice how fluid and light your gait has become. Notice also if you feel more balance as you walk.

PART 2: "PIERRE DE WIESSANT"

1. Return to "The Thinker" position. This time allow your hand to come forward as your elbow comes forward. Thus, instead of just your elbow, you are now presenting your entire forearm to the imaginary pad.

A. Go back and forth several times, each time tapping the imaginary pad with your entire forearm. Move the pad to the right and left, noticing how your chest, shoulder, hip, and foot respond with each directional change. Pause.

---

[34] Note that some of the basic movements in *shuaijiao*, Bagua, and other martial arts also exhibit similar, though obviously not identical, mechanics. For example, the sequences in *kai* from *shuaijiao* and Bagua, *uki waza* and *yoko guruma* in judo, and Grasping Sparrow's Tail and Fair Lady Works Shuttle from Taichi require a similar connection of the legs, pelvis, and spine. The typical break-fall in response to *kotogaeshi* in aikido is one possible continuation of such spiraling, where the rotation of metacarpals in concert with flexion of the wrist leads the movement of the spine and pelvis, rather than vice versa. For a nice example of uppercuts, see: Precision Striking, "Boxer Uppercut Tips: 5 Common Errors, Part 1 of 3," YouTube, October 11, 2017, https://youtu.be/GBRRy905Q2Q.

B. Go back and forth several times.

C. Rest.

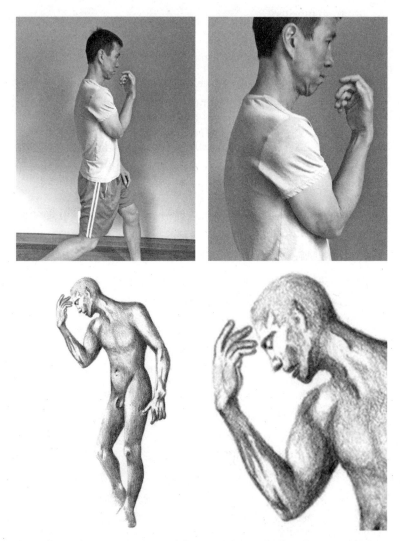

Steps 2 and 3, and a close-up of "Pierre de Wiessant hand" (pencil rendition of *Pierre de Wiessant* by Andreia de Abreu Gomes).

2. Resume the previous movement, and this time spiral your fist in a *counterclockwise* direction as your forearm comes forward. You can pretend that you have a message written on the back of your hand and you want to display it to someone standing to your left. (If you are on the opposite side with your left forearm striking the imaginary pad, your left fist will spiral in the opposite direction; in this case, clockwise.)

   A. Notice how the spiraling of your hand accentuates every aspect of the movement all the way down to your feet.

   B. Go back and forth a few times and begin to freeze at the end of the movement. (In this position you will bear some resemblance to another of Rodin's sculptures.)[35]

   C. Repeat several times slowly, coordinating the spiraling of your fist with the movement of your elbow, hip, and foot.

   D. Rest.

3. Repeat the previous step but begin to speed up the motion at the end.

   A. Go back and forth, slowing down anytime you want to improve your precision.

   B. Every now and then, freeze at the end of the motion and check the positioning of different parts of yourself.

   C. Once again, have fun with the movement. (And if the spiraling of your hand feels like it's too distracting at any moment, leave it out.)

   D. Rest whenever you want. When you are ready, walk around and feel the difference in your gait. The two sides will probably feel very different from each other. Notice which shoulder you lead with when you walk. Which arm feels longer? Which hip feels more open?

4. Repeat all the steps on the opposite side (with your right leg forward). When you are finished, notice how fluid and light your gait has become. Notice also if you feel more fluid and powerful as you walk.

---

[35] *Pierre de Wiessant.* See https://tinyurl.com/uwvw94c for a photograph of the sculpture.

Lesson 25
Resistance as a Learning Tool[36]

(Make sure you have completed the previous four lessons before starting this one.)

The sensory feedback provided by lightly touching or tapping a target can help to guide your movement. Increased physical resistance provides additional sensory feedback such that it can, if applied judiciously, help you to improve economy of motion. If applied indiscriminately, on the other hand, resistance will more likely subvert learning and lead you to develop bad habits.

PART 1: MAKING CONTACT WITH YOUR ELBOW (TO BE EXPLORED WITH A PARTNER HOLDING A MITT OR ALONE WITH A HEAVY BAG)

Starting Position: "The Thinker" position (from the end of Part I, Lesson 24).

1. Repeat some of the final movements of the previous lesson, where you are flicking your right elbow forward to tap an imaginary pad. For now, keep your right hand against the right side of your jaw.

   A. Play with a few flicks before freezing at the end of your motion.

   B. Have a partner hold a pad or boxing mitt where your elbow ends. Continue flicking your elbow, allowing it to hit the mitt. Your partner can accentuate the feedback by slapping the pad lightly into your elbow as your elbow comes forward.

   C. For variety, you can have your partner place the pad in different locations (farther to the right or farther to the left) on each iteration. Note that each location should subtly alter the way you use your entire body.

---

[36] Both Lessons 24 and 25 provide a nice complement to step 6 of Lesson 17, "Reach and Roll on Your Back."

D. If you don't have a partner, you can play with this same motion on a heavy bag. Take your time to carefully line yourself up with the bag before flicking. (Some bags are quite hard and abrasive on the outside, so you may want to tape your elbow or wear padding over it before trying this.)

E. Slow down from time to time so that you can check the precision of your movement from head to toe, and metacarpal to metatarsal.

F. Rest after playing for a bit. (I recommend not turning this into a workout until you've gotten more proficient at the movement.)

2. Resume again, but this time allow your hand to leave your chin so that your entire forearm comes forward. Begin to tap the pad with your entire forearm.

A. Keep the movement light.

B. Go back and forth several times before resting.

3. Repeat all the steps on the other side.

PART 2: MAKING CONTACT WITH YOUR KNUCKLES (TO BE EXPLORED WITH A PARTNER HOLDING A PAD)

1. Resume the final movements from part 1 of this lesson. Freeze at the very end of your movement and notice where your fist ends up. This time, have your partner very lightly hold a pad (facing downward) where your fist ends.

A. Begin to repeat the entire motion slowly, each time ending with your fist against the pad.

B. Play with having the weight of your back foot on different metatarsals. (If you have a weak and vulnerable ankle, simply stay closer to the 1st and 2nd metatarsals.) Make sure you are not leaning forward. Allow your elbow to reach forward at the end.

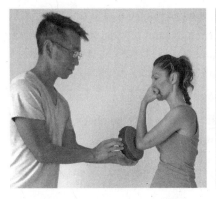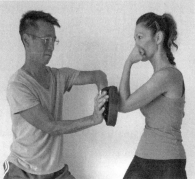

The elbow taps the pad lightly (left) or with more force (right). In the preliminary stage, keep your knuckles connected to your face.

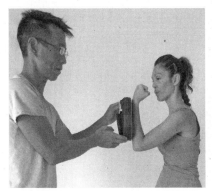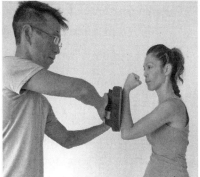

Forearm taps pad lightly (left) or with more force (right).

C. Gradually increase the speed at the very end. Make sure your partner is holding the pad very lightly (preferably with the fingertips) so that it pops up when you hit it. Do not attempt to hit hard. Keep the movement easy and light. Eventually, you will find yourself simply flicking your back foot and simultaneously flicking both your right hip and your right elbow forward.

D. As the flicking gets faster, you will find your fist tapping the pad with increased velocity. Once again, do not try to hit with great force, just focus on making the movement light and easy.

E. It is important to slow your movements down dramatically whenever you find yourself getting off target. Either way, slow down from time to time so that you can check the precision of your movement from head to toe, and metacarpal to metatarsal. Allow both the feel of tapping the pad and the sound it makes help to guide your movement.

F. Once again, I don't recommend turning this into a workout—at least not until you've gotten more proficient at the movements.

G. Rest after several iterations.

2. Walk around and compare your two sides before repeating any or all of the steps on the opposite side (with your right foot forward).

PART 3: MORE RESISTANCE (USING WRAPS AND GLOVES)

Because there is a slightly higher risk for injury to your hand, wrist, and shoulder in this part of the lesson, I recommend you do the following:

- Find a partner who has experience using mitts and wrapping hands, or alternatively watch a YouTube video on how to wrap them yourself.[37]

- After wrapping your hands, put on a pair of boxing gloves.

- As always, proceed slowly so that you can attend to your own movements and thereby increase your level of accuracy and precision while reducing the risk of injuring yourself or your partner.

1. Repeat the final movements of part 2 and freeze at the end of your trajectory (with your elbow forward and your fist at its highest point).

A. Have your partner press down with a pad very gently into your fist.

---

[37] The YouTube channel called Precision Striking has a nice one called "How to Wrap Your Hands for Boxing: Protect Your Hands for the Long Run," February 3, 2018, https://youtu.be/mSxW47G0_NI.

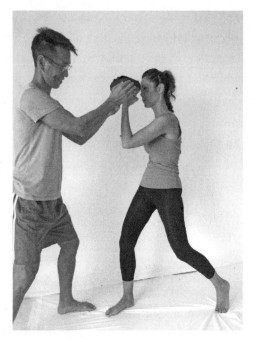

Light tapping with fist.

B. Your wrist should be somewhat rigid and straight at this point. Try adjusting your hand and wrist so that the mitt is pressing into your first two knuckles.

C. Have your partner increase pressure gradually and see if you can maintain a firm wrist. If you feel your wrist weakening, stop immediately.

D. As your partner increases pressure, you will feel where in your body you are not connected—where, in other words, there are weak links in the chain between your fist and your feet.

E. Ask your partner to let off on the pressure whenever you start to feel collapsing in some part of your body and find ways to make small adjustments in order to remedy the situation. In this manner you will refine the positioning of everything from your hand down to your foot.

2. Once you feel comfortable with the previous steps, return to rotating your body back and forth slowly, gradually picking up speed. This time have your partner gently slap the mitt downward as your glove rises upward.

   A. As you gradually pick up speed and your glove rises with more force, have your partner slap down a little harder. Make sure your partner increases the downward force *gradually* and not all at once so that your body, and particularly your shoulder, can get used to the increasing resistance. The gradualness will also allow your partner to get used to the increasing force.

   B. At some point, the upward force of the glove meeting the downward force of the mitt will make a resounding pop.

   C. Stop to make adjustments as needed.

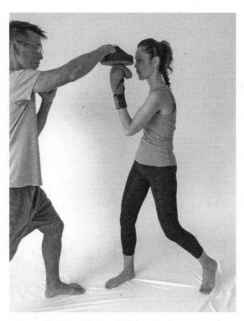

Gradually increase resistance and velocity. Stop frequently to check your positioning and make the necessary adjustments.

Lesson 26
Improving Circulation

One of my favorite lessons in this book, "Improving Circulation" will help you get a clearer feeling for how your spine and rib cage can assist in powerfully driving your feet and knees during all phases of your stride, thereby acting as a "turbocharger" of sorts.[38] As an added bonus, this lesson could help with your hitch-kick if, in addition to being a runner, you happen to be a long-jumper.

Starting Position: Lie on your right side with your right knee bent in front of you and your left knee bent and resting somewhere behind it. (For those who are not so flexible, don't worry if your left knee doesn't reach the floor.) Place your left palm on the floor in front of you with your left arm in a push-up position. Have your right arm relatively straight and pointing at a downward angle. If you feel any discomfort in your neck or right shoulder, cradle your head with your right arm or fold some towels neatly and place them under your head.

1. Begin to gently pull your right knee upward toward your chest. The entire weight of your body is on your right side, so I don't recommend muscling your knee all the way to your chest. Instead, allow the movement to remain tiny and discover how the rest of your body *responds* to the pulling. In this sense it will feel as if you are pulling your chest toward your knee rather than vice versa.

   A. Pull gently, and then reverse the motion and slowly push your right knee away from your chest—or, if you prefer, gently push your chest away from your knee.

   B. As you pull upward and downward you will feel your chest and even your neck moving.

   C. When you pull your knee upward, can you feel yourself getting shorter? When you push it downward, can you feel yourself getting taller?

---

[38] This lesson is inspired in part by Frank Wildman's "Pelvis Is the Core of Strength" workshop, given in New York City between 2002 and 2004, and his "Modigliani Legs" lesson, recorded at an unknown public workshop. (Thanks to my colleague Ellen Gordon for so generously sharing a tape of "Modigliani Legs" with me back in 2004.)

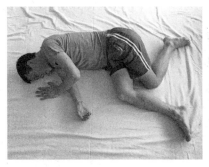
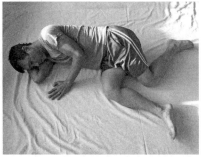

Left: without the bottom arm supporting the head. Right: with the bottom arm supporting the head.

D. Go back and forth very slowly, noticing what is happening in your trunk.

E. Rest.

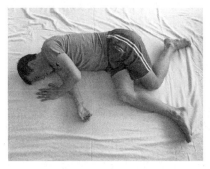
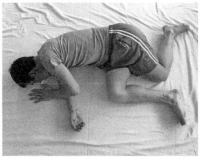

Neutral position (left) versus sliding the right knee (the front knee) upward (right). Notice how my torso responds to the movement of my leg by rolling toward the floor. Notice also how my opposite leg (the back leg) responds.

2. Resume the previous position, and this time, begin to trace a circle on the floor with your right ankle. Make it as small or as large as you want.

A. Notice that in order to make truer circles, your knee will have to slide a little on the floor.

B. Feel how your chest is involved in the movement. Once again, you will feel yourself getting taller and shorter.

C. What is happening with your opposite foot? What about your opposite knee?

D. After a few circles, reverse the direction.

E. After one or two circles in this direction, reverse again.

F. Rest on your back and feel the difference between your two sides.

3. Resume the previous exploration and observe how your opposite leg responds.

A. Can you feel how the opposite leg assists in making the circles possible? Can you feel the movement reverberating in your chest and even in your neck?

B. If you pay close attention, you'll notice that your left foot is also making a circle, but one that is out of phase with that made by your right foot. How far out of phase is your left foot—in other words, how far does it lag behind in drawing its own circle?

C. In order for the movement to be easier and more efficient, one foot must be lagging no more and no less than a certain amount. Experiment to see if you can discover what amount of lagging gives you more, and what amount gives you less, ease in the movement.

D. Rest after a while.

4. Resume the previous exploration. Continue searching for the proper amount of lag in your foot in back.

A. To generate the greatest amount of power, thereby allowing you to expend the least amount of energy, your two feet should be exactly 180 degrees out of phase. This means when your right foot is moving in an upward arc, your left foot is moving in a downward arc, and vice versa. At any given moment, your right and left foot should be on the exact opposite sides of their respective circles, as when you are riding a bicycle.

B. Does this motion remind you of anything? Have you ever felt any of these sensations in your body while running? Can you sense how this could be a useful exploration for the long jump?

C. Slow down to get a sense of exactly how the movement of your left foot assists the movement of your right foot and vice versa. If the movement of your feet is not precisely synchronized—that is, if they are moving even a little out of phase—you will find the movement to be more difficult and thus more of an effort.

D. If you get confused, slow down, reduce the size of the movement, and search for how one side can *respond* to the other.

E. After a few circles, reverse the direction.

F. Don't force anything. Simply search for the feeling of harmony in your body. If you cannot find it, keep slowing down, or simply stop and rest for a while. Remember that you can always quit for a while and come back to the lesson at some later date.

G. After a few circles in this direction, rest on your back and notice what is different in your breathing.

5. Resume the previous position and continue making circles with your right foot. This time keep your head lifted off the floor as you make circles.

A. Keeping your head off the floor will help to accentuate rolling over your right shoulder as you go through your circles.

B. As long as you are not unnecessarily tensing your left shoulder (your top shoulder), it will make circles, or some sort of oval, too. Even your elbow is "circulating." Your entire body can, in fact, be involved in the circulating.

C. Do you feel yourself getting taller and shorter during different phases of the circle?

D. Begin to make the movement larger and larger.

E. Feel how much your trunk is involved.

F. Begin to speed up the movement.

G. After a few iterations, gradually slow down and make the movement smaller.

H. What does this motion remind you of?

I. Rest on your back when you are ready.

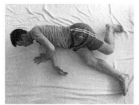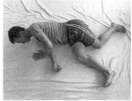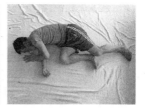

Keeping my head up and making fairly large circles with my right foot (the front foot). From right to left, notice how I get progressively taller and how my left leg (the back leg) is also making circles.

6. Resume the previous exploration and begin to observe the movement of your left hand. How does it move in conjunction with the movement of your right knee?

A. If you are very attentive, you will notice that your hand is tracing circles on the floor.

B. At some point, place the back of your left hand on the floor.

C. Observe how the weight rolls over different metacarpals as you continue to make circles with your knee.

D. Reverse the direction of circle-making and continue to observe.

E. Rest whenever you want to.

7. This time place your left leg in front of your right leg. (In this position, your bottom leg is behind and your top leg is in front.) Have both knees slightly bent.

A. Begin to slide your right foot closer to your buttocks and then slide it back. Feel the response in your chest. As your right foot moves closer to your buttocks, you will feel your trunk rolling forward toward the floor.

B. Go back and forth, seeing how close you can bring your foot to your buttocks without straining.

C. Pause.

8. Once again bring your foot as close as you can to your buttocks. When your foot is in this position, begin to pull your right knee toward your chest and then gently push it away.

A. Because your right leg is pinned to the floor, it won't slide much, if at all, unless you strain. Allow the movement to stay small and observe how your left leg begins to move backward and downward in response. You will feel your thighs rubbing against each other. Though your initial focus was to pull or push your right knee (back knee), your left leg (top leg) is the one that should be more obviously in motion.

B. Very slowly go back and forth. Begin to minimize your effort. Notice how much movement there is in your chest.

C. Begin to make the movement larger and faster. If you get confused, slow down again.

D. Rest when you feel like it.

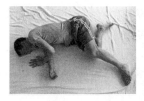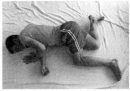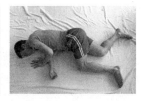

With right leg behind: neutral (right), bringing right heel toward buttock (middle), right knee toward chest (left). Notice how the front leg responds.

9. Begin to make circles with your back foot.

    A. Notice how your opposite foot and leg respond.

    B. If your feet stay on opposite sides of their respective circles, meaning that they are moving exactly 180 degrees out of phase, you will feel a good deal of power. If this is not happening, slow down the movement and make it much smaller again until you can bring them in synchrony such that they are 180 degrees out of phase.

    C. Observe the movement of your head. Experiment with having it on the floor and lifted off the floor. Is it making circles?

    D. Gradually increase the size and speed of the motion. Notice how much your chest and head are moving.

    E. Gradually decrease the size and speed until you come to a rest.

    F. Rest on your back.

10. Repeat all the steps facing the other side, then walk around and notice how smooth, light, and powerful your gait has become. Does your chest feel like it's floating? Run down the block to see if you can identify any of the sensations that you had on the floor in your stride.

11. Optional Step 1: Lie on either side with the bottom leg in front. Begin to make small circles with your front foot.

    A. Just as before, sense the involvement of your chest and head. Notice what your opposite foot and opposite knee are doing.

    B. See to it that your feet are 180 degrees out of phase.

    C. Gradually increase the size of the circle. As it gets larger you will feel both knees moving more. You will feel your head and chest going up and down. (You have the option of lifting your head or letting it roll or slide on the floor.)

    D. At some point when the circle gets large enough, you will feel your legs wanting to pass each other: the top leg will move to the front and the bottom leg will move to the back.

E. Continue increasing the size, and each leg will begin to alternate between being in front and being in back.

F. Keep the movement slow so that you can more clearly feel how your chest and head respond to the movement.

G. Gradually decrease the movement until the legs are no longer alternating sides. Diminish the circles until they are very tiny, then rest.

12. Optional Step 2: Repeat the previous step facing to the opposite side.

Lesson 27

Where Does My Arm Begin?
(Reach and Roll on Your Side)[39]

Starting Position: Lie on your right side and draw your knees up toward your chest such that your thighs make a 90-degree angle with your torso. Have your right arm straight out in front of you and rest your left hand comfortably on top of the right. Notice the texture of your right hand.

1. Begin to slide your left hand forward a little, exploring the feeling of your right hand beneath it. Then slide your hand back to where it started. Go back and forth very slowly, each time trying to make the movement easier and less effortful. Ask yourself, "Where does my arm begin?" As you continue the movement, you may find yourself reaching beyond your right hand. This is not so much a goal as a possibility. How could it happen?

A. Notice what is moving besides your hand. For example, what is your elbow doing? Your left shoulder? What about your head? Do the movement with your eyes closed and notice if your head begins to turn. Could the movement of your head have any connection with the movement of your hand?

B. After exploring the movement several times, rest on your back.

---

[39] For another take on some of the rotational concepts in this lesson, go to Lesson 2, "Screwing Foot into Wall," or Lesson 17, "Reach and Roll on Your Back."

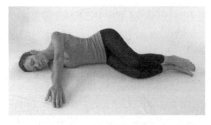 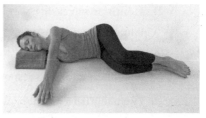

You can choose to go without support (left), or if it's more comfortable, with firm support under your head (right).

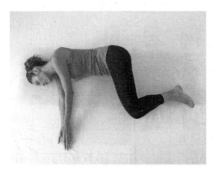 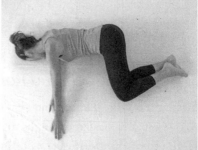

Bird's-eye view.

2. Roll over to the same side and come to the same position. Now begin to slide your left hand back so that you can feel the contour of your right wrist, forearm, and eventually the crook of your right elbow. While you do this, keep your left elbow relatively straight. Note that keeping the left elbow straight does not require that you lock the elbow (in fact, locking it will probably be less comfortable). It may seem difficult or even impossible to slide the hand very far while the elbow stays fairly straight.

    A. Could moving some other part of your body make the movement possible?

    B. For the next minute or two, continue searching for ways to slide your hand backward without bending the elbow. If you are still wondering how to do it, continue wondering, knowing that wondering is far more important than "getting it right"; maybe there is no "right."

C. Give yourself permission to forget about the lesson and do something else altogether. If you choose to continue with the lesson, rest on your back for a few moments before continuing.

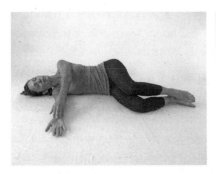 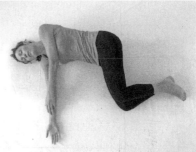

Side view (left) and bird's eye view (right) of step 2.

3. Roll over to the same side and come to the same position, and once again wonder where your left arm begins. Let go of the first answer that comes to mind. Then let go of the second. And the third. Slide your left hand forward and then bring it back to where it was initially resting. Go back and forth several times before pausing.

   A. Imagine there is a button directly in front of your left knee and that you want to push it. Reach forward gently with your left knee to push the button. Note that forward, in this case, does not mean toward your chest. In addition, keep in mind that you don't need to lift your leg—in other words, it can stay in contact with the other leg—and you don't need to lift your ankle.

   B. Go slowly so that you can really feel what is happening. Each time you slide the knee forward, and then back to neutral, notice what's happening in your left hip. Is there movement in your back? Is your left shoulder moving at all? What could be preventing your knee from moving farther (without exerting more effort)? Again, note that it doesn't matter whether or not your knee moves farther or whether you "get it right." Possibly what matters the most is knowing that it doesn't matter. Rest on your back.

4. Roll over to the same position. Slide both your left knee and left
hand forward at the same time. If there were a mirror in front of
you, your hand would be reaching toward the hand in the mirror
and your knee toward the knee in the mirror. Try to move hand
and knee in total synchrony so that one does not go faster than the
other. Go slowly enough so that you notice when one or the other
begins to get ahead.

A. Go forward and then back to neutral several times slowly,
noticing when the movement is not so smooth. Cut your speed
down to one-fifth of the original. This means really slow down.
(One trick I use for myself is to measure time: if it originally
took me one second to complete the movement, then one-
fifth the speed would mean completing the movement in five
seconds.)

B. Try leading the movement once with your knee, and then
once with your hand—alternate back and forth several times.
Notice how leading with a different part changes the movement. Pause.

C. Slide your left hand forward and back to neutral. Notice if
the movement has gotten easier and that you are able to reach
farther without any strain. Even if the movement doesn't feel
easier, trust that over time—perhaps not today—it will. From a
neurological perspective, things have already begun to change as
a result of your slow exploration.

D. Lie on your back. Notice how one leg feels much longer than
the other. You may feel that one arm also feels longer. It may
feel like the floor is tilting to the right or left. This means
that excessive muscle tension has just disappeared from half
of your body, allowing that half to rest more fully into the
floor. If you really pay attention, you will notice that half
of you is expanding more as you inhale. This is because you
have actually increased the breathing capacity in half of
your body.

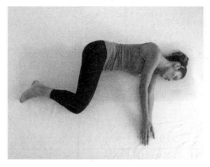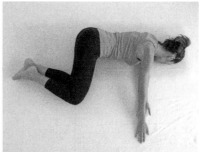

Bird's-eye view: Notice how Raquel's head follows the movement of her right arm as it reaches forward.

5. Roll over to the same side. Slide your left knee backward—as if the button now pushes back into your knee. Slide back and return to neutral several times. Notice if your back and shoulder are moving along with your knee. You may find your left hand sliding backward automatically. Go back and forth a few times before pausing.

A. As you slide your knee backward, intentionally slide your left hand backward while keeping your elbow relatively straight. See if you can slide the two in complete synchrony. Be lazy so that you minimize effort. For example, see if you can slide your arm without tensing your shoulder. Go back and forth a few times before pausing.

B. Now simply slide your hand backward (still keeping your elbow relatively straight). Can you feel your back and rib cage turning with you? Go back and forth a few times slowly before pausing.

C. Now slide your knee backward. What parts of your body are moving besides your knee? Go back and forth several times with your knee, sensing what else is moving.

D. Now slide both knee and hand all the way forward and all the way backward. Note that at some point in going backward, your knee will begin to lift automatically without effort. Allow it to do so. Close your eyes. As you slide forward, allow your head to turn so that your nose comes toward the floor. As you slide backward, allow your head to turn so that your nose begins to point toward the ceiling. Go back and forth several times slowly, paying attention so that your neck stays soft and comfortable and that your head turns only as far as is extremely comfortable.

E. Pause and simply slide your hand forward and backward, keeping your eyes closed. Has the movement gotten easier? Once again, ask yourself, "I wonder where my arm begins?" Rest on your back and notice how different the right and left sides of your body feel. One side is resting much more into the floor because parasitic tension has left that side. One might even say that you have increased the flow of qi on that side.

6. Repeat steps 1 to 5 lying on your other side.

7. When you are finished, both sides will feel more even, and you may find that your whole body is sinking more into the floor. Now a great deal of parasitic tension has left both sides of the body.

8. Take your time to slowly roll over and stand up. Close your eyes and feel how open your chest has become and how much lower your shoulders are resting. Do you feel taller? Are you more grounded in your feet? Does your chest feel like it's floating? All of these remarkable changes have occurred through slowing down, wondering, and observing. You have dissolved parasitic tension while simultaneously awakening dormant parts of yourself. Take a few moments to savor this feeling. Then open your eyes and take a walk, noticing how different walking feels.

Acknowledgments

It is difficult to have firsts and lasts when talking about people who have made writing and eventually publishing this book possible, but linear space-time requires order, so here goes.... Thank you to my wife, Andreia, my closest confidant and teacher of all the important things in life. Your patience and support have played an invaluable role in making all of this possible. Thanks also to my parents and my sister Ann, for your unwavering support and encouragement.

A big thanks to Elizabeth Beringer for providing crucial support over the years. Thanks also to David Zemach-Bersin, Tim McKee, Elizabeth (again), and Carol Kress for making this publication possible, and to John Cedric Tarr and Carey Benom for taking the time to review the Postscript and to give insightful comments.

A deep bow to Master Xueyi Li and Master Guoliang Ge for playing a pivotal role in getting me to slow down and pay attention. Without your painstaking guidance, I would probably never have discovered what it really means to learn. Thanks also to Shimu Li and Shimu Ge (in Chinese, *shimu* can be used in reference to the wife of one's master). Where Master Li and Master Ge have provided me with fatherly love and guidance during my time in China, Shimu Li and Shimu Ge have shown me motherly warmth and a soft complement to the masters' old-school ways.

Another deep bow to Master Don Schule and Pengfu Yuan: your teachings on martial arts and life have left a deep and lasting impression.

A big shout out to John Cedric Tarr, Göran Mörkeberg, and José Agustín Candisano for many thought-provoking and inspiring conversations and letters related to learning, Feldenkrais, running, fitness, and the industries that surround them. Your support provided not only intellectual stimulation but a boost to morale during recent lean times.

Kudos to Frank Wildman for bringing ingenuity into the teaching of the Feldenkrais Method. I have lifted many ideas from you and brought them into both my teaching and writing (some of them appear in this book).

Hats off to Ruthy Alon, for providing me with a rich new context for lessons in your Bones for Life training. (Thanks also to Ellen Gordon and Gretchen Langer for so generously introducing me to Ruthy.)

Thank you Jeff Haller for generously taking the time to share new and important perspectives on fitness, Taichi, martial arts, and, of course, Feldenkrais. Thanks also, Robbie Ofir, for your generosity, empathy, and integrity in assisting in the New York Feldenkrais Training.

Thanks to Chuck Eisenstein, whose ideas have influenced much of my writing over the years.

Thanks also to Emily Simon and Sally Searles for giving me the precious opportunity of teaching my first running classes in Ann Arbor, back in '04, to Ellen Gordon for helping me choose the lessons for my first running workshop (also in Ann Arbor in '04), and to Gisela Forero Burquet, Ned Liebl, Carolin Theuring, Terrence Mahon, Al Wadleigh, Alex Maslansky, and Stories Bookstore for continued support.

I owe a great debt to the following people, who played a pivotal role in my development in martial arts and Feldenkrais: my first martial arts teachers, Yin Xie and Ying Shui, who attempted to teach this old (and stiff) dog new tricks; Dogo (Stephen Backaus), who introduced me to Feldenkrais back in '94 and lent me the book on the subject that would change the course of my life; Master Wuxing Chen and Victor Kan, who so generously shared some of their knowledge on Chen-style Taichi with me; Bruce Ching, for brief but vital guidance in Taichi stances; Larry and Maya Spence, Boyan Brodaric, Gail Macdonald, Jim Eisenstein, Marilyn Shoboken, and Avis Jones, all of whom braved my first Feldenkrais classes; Tony Lasbeur at DTLA Fight Club, Hide at Ktown Boxing Club, and Joseph Del Real at California Kickboxing, each of whom separately gave me a good reality check and generously taught as much about the pugilistic arts as this beginner could absorb in a short period; all of my Bagua "uncles" and "brothers" in Tianjin who generously taught me and welcomed me into the lineage; Peter Woolf and Leeann Fu, who continue to share important insights on learning and life; Cheryl Herzog, who generously provided me with my first Functional Integration lesson—a lovely introduction to the Feldenkrais Method; Al and Avis Jones, who so generously shared their time, expertise, and labor in a joint project to construct my first Feldenkrais folding table; and Professor Ken Knott, who kindly introduced me to judo great Trevor Leggett.

Finally, thank you to all of my students, along with all of the people who have given me teaching opportunities—unknowingly, you have provided a vast space for me to learn and grow.

Attributions for Quotations

page xii: Terry Gilliam, introduction to a screening of the 2005 film *Tideland*.

page 1: Margaret Mead, *Male and Female: A Study of the Sexes in a Changing World*, 19.

page 7: Andre Agassi, *Open: An Autobiography*, 1.

page 8: Trevor Leggett, *The Dragon Mask*, www.bestjudo.com (go to https://tinyurl .com/yxy2csll and scroll down to the story titled "Training").

page 11: Alan Watts, *The Culture of Counter Culture: The Edited Transcripts*, 58.

page 12: Ari Weinzweig, *Zingerman's Guide to Good Eating*, 400.

page 15: Josh Waitzkin, *The Art of Learning: A Journey in the Pursuit of Excellence*, 186–87.

page 19: James Gleick, *Isaac Newton*, 38.

page 23: Albert Einstein, quoted in "Einstein Revealed," broadcast on PBS's *Nova* in 1999. According to producer Thomas Levenson (personal correspondence): "That quote was a collage of a couple of different Einstein aphorisms, I believe sourced from Alice Calaprice's *The Quotable Einstein*. In that documentary we operated under two rules: if the actor playing Einstein was speaking on camera, we would rewrite Einstein's original words as needed to transform written expression into speakable lines. If quoted in voice-over, without seeing the actor's lips move, those quotes were exact [translations]."

page 26: Keith Johnstone, *Improvisation and the Theatre*, 80.

page 29: Magda Gerber, *Dear Infant: Caring for Infants with Respect*, 64.

page 35: Stanley Keleman, *Your Body Speaks Its Mind*, 37–38.

page 38: Alan Watts, "A Cure for Education," excerpted in *Mountains are Mountains and Rivers are Rivers*, 27–28.

page 40: Don Hanlon Johnson, *Body: Recovering Our Sensual Wisdom*, 81.

page 47: Andre Agassi, *Open: An Autobiography*, 1.

page 49: David Graeber, *Bullshit Jobs: A Theory*, 13.

page 51: Moshe Feldenkrais (one of the many sayings attributed to him by his students).

page 53: W. Timothy Gallwey, *The Inner Game of Tennis*, 148.

page 54: Charles Eisenstein, *Yoga of Eating,* public lecture in Philadelphia, 2007.

page 61: Dave Barry, *Miami Herald,* December 1, 1996.

page 77: Thomas Hanna, *Body of Life: Creating New Pathways for Sensory Awareness and Fluid Movement,* 38.

page 85: Jared Diamond, *The World Until Yesterday: What Can We Learn from Traditional Societies?* 8–9.

page 93: Thomas Hauser, *Muhammad Ali: His Life and Times,* 19.

page 93: Dave Lowry, *Traditions: Essays on the Japanese Martial Arts and Ways,* 144.

page 96: Ellen Langer, *On Becoming an Artist,* 151.

page 109: Otto Pohl, "Improving the Way Humans Walk," *New York Times,* March 12, 2002.

page 113: Rene Lynch, "Skechers Lawsuit: How to Get Your Piece of the $40-Million Payout," *Los Angeles Times,* May 17, 2012.

page 117: John O'Neil, "Vital Signs: Protection; Textured Insoles Win High Scores," *New York Times,* April 8, 2003.

page 123: Jess O'Brien, editor, *Nei Jia Quan: Internal Martial Arts,* 165.

page 129: Thomas Merton, in a letter to Jim Forest dated February 21, 1966, reproduced in *Hidden Ground of Love: The Letters of Thomas Merton on Religious Experience and Social Concerns,* 1993.

page 131: Deane Juhan, *Job's Body,* 253.

page 135: Charles Eisenstein, "Mutiny of the Soul," *Reality Sandwich,* October 7, 2008.

page 139: Carl Sagan, *The Varieties of Scientific Experience,* 90.

page 143: Fritjof Capra, *Hidden Connections,* 126.

page 147: Erich Schiffmann, *Yoga,* 3–4.

page 150: Stanley Keleman, *Your Body Speaks Its Mind,* 63.

page 152: Thomas Hanna, *Body of Life,* 34.

page 153: Joseph Campbell, *Reflections on the Art of Living: A Joseph Campbell Companion,* 26.

page 156: Wolfe Lowenthal, *There Are No Secrets,* 40.

page 159: Noam Chomsky, *Chomsky on Mis-Education,* 38.

page 181: Moshe Feldenkrais, *The Elusive Obvious,* 150.

page 182: Robert W. Smith, *Martial Musings,* 205.

page 184: W. Timothy Gallwey, *Inner Tennis,* 169.

Bibliography

Agassi, Andre. *Open: An Autobiography.* New York: Alfred A. Knopf, 2009.

Alon, Ruthy. *Mindful Spontaneity: Lessons in the Feldenkrais Method.* Berkeley, CA: North Atlantic Books, 1996.

Barry, Dave. "Classic '96: King of the Road." *Miami Herald.* December 1, 1996.

Brennan, Danielle, "Olympian Michael Johnson on How He Learned to Love His 'Funny' Upright Running Style." *Today,* July 13, 2016.

Campbell, Joseph. *Reflections on the Art of Living: A Joseph Campbell Companion.* Edited by Diane K. Osbon. New York: Harper Perennial, 1998.

Capra, Fritjof. *Hidden Connections.* New York: Anchor, 2004.

Castaño, J. D. *"Tideland:* Terry Gilliam Intro Subtitulado." Video. November 30, 2011. Web. 11 Sep. 2018. https://youtu.be/bPiC0FQSiWY.

Chomsky, Noam. *Chomsky on Mis-Education.* Edited by Donaldo Macedo. Lanham, MD: Rowman & Littlefield, 2004.

Cranz, Galen. *The Chair: Rethinking Culture, Body & Design.* New York: W. W. Norton, 1998.

Damasio, Antonio. *The Feeling of What Happens.* New York: Mariner, 2000.

Diamond, Jared. *The World Until Yesterday: What Can We Learn from Traditional Societies?* New York: Penguin, 2012.

Dreyer, Danny, and Katherine Dreyer. *ChiRunning: A Revolutionary Approach to Effortless, Injury-Free Running.* New York: Fireside, 2009.

Dychtwald, Ken. *Bodymind.* New York: Pantheon, 1977.

Eisenstein, Charles. "Mutiny of the Soul." *Reality Sandwich,* October 7, 2008.

Eisenstein, Charles. *Sacred Economics: Money, Gift and Society in the Age of Transition.* Berkeley, CA: North Atlantic Books, 2011.

Eisenstein, Charles. *The Yoga of Eating.* Public lecture in Philadelphia, 2007.

Feldenkrais, Moshe. *Awareness through Movement.* New York: Harper-Collins, 1990.

Feldenkrais, Moshe. *Body and Mature Behavior: A Study of Anxiety, Sex, Gravitation & Learning.* Madison, CT: International Universities Press, 1992.

Feldenkrais, Moshe. *The Elusive Obvious: The Convergence of Movement, Neuroplasticity and Health.* Berkeley, CA: North Atlantic Books and Somatic Resources, 2019.

Gallwey, W. Timothy. *The Inner Game of Tennis.* New York: Random House, 1974.

Gallwey, W. Timothy. *Inner Tennis: Playing the Game.* New York: Random House, 1976.

Gerber, Magda. *Dear Infant: Caring for Infants With Respect.* Edited by Joan Weaver. Los Angeles: Resources for Infant Educare (RIE), 2002.

Gilliam, Terry, director. *Tideland.* Film. Recorded Picture Co., 2006.

Gleick, James. *Isaac Newton.* New York: Pantheon, 2003.

Gleick, James. *Genius: The Life and Science of Richard Feynman.* New York: Pantheon, 1992.

Graeber, David. *Bullshit Jobs: A Theory.* New York: Penguin, 2018.

Hanna, Thomas. *Body of Life: Creating New Pathways for Sensory Awareness and Fluid Movement.* Rochester, VT: Healing Arts Press, 1979.

Hari, Johann. *Chasing the Scream: The First and Last Days of the War on Drugs.* New York: Bloomsbury, 2019.

Hari, Johann. *Lost Connections: Uncovering the Real Causes of Depression—and the Unexpected Solutions.* New York: Bloomsbury, 2018.

Hauser, Thomas. *Muhammad Ali: His Life and Times.* New York: Simon & Schuster, 1991.

Hochschild, Arlie. *The Managed Heart: Commercialization of Human Feeling.* Berkeley, CA: University of California Press, 2012.

Hudson, Michael. *And Forgive Them Their Debts: Lending, Foreclosure and Redemption from Bronze Age Finance to the Jubilee Year.* Dresden, Germany: ISLET, 2018.

Johnson, Don Hanlon. *Body: Recovering Our Sensual Wisdom.* Berkeley, CA: North Atlantic Books, 1992.

Johnstone, Keith. *Improvisation and the Theatre.* New York: Routledge/Theatre Arts, 1992.

Juhan, Deane. *Job's Body.* Barrytown, NY: Barrytown/Station Hill Press, 2003.

Keen, Mary. "Early Development and Attainment of Normal Mature Gait," *Journal of Prosthetics and Orthotics* 5:2 (April 1993), 37/25.

Keleman, Stanley. *Your Body Speaks Its Mind.* Berkeley, CA: Center Press, 1981.

Lakoff, George. *Moral Politics: What Conservatives Know That Liberals Don't.* Chicago: University of Chicago Press, 1996.

Langer, Ellen. *On Becoming an Artist.* New York: Ballantine, 2005.

Leggett, Trevor. *The Dragon Mask.* London: Ippon, 1995.

Lenzen, Manuela. "Feeling Our Emotions." *Scientific American Mind,* April 14–15, 2005.

Lowenthal, Wolfe. *There Are No Secrets: Professor Cheng Man-ch'ing and His Tai Chi Chuan.* Berkeley, CA: North Atlantic Books, 1991.

Lowry, Dave. *Traditions: Essays on the Japanese Martial Arts and Ways.* Boston: Tuttle, 2002.

Lyle, Stephen, and Leon Mann, directors. *Usain Bolt: The Fastest Man Who Has Ever Lived.* BBC 2 Television, May 15, 2010.

Mead, Margaret. *Male and Female: A Study of the Sexes in a Changing World.* New York: William Morrow, 1955.

Merton, Thomas. *Hidden Ground of Love: The Letters of Thomas Merton on Religious Experience and Social Concerns.* Edited by William H. Shannon. New York: Farrar, Straus and Giroux, 1985.

O'Brien, Jess, editor. *Nei Jia Quan: Internal Martial Arts.* Berkeley, CA: North Atlantic Books, 2004.

O'Neil, John. "Protection: Textured Soles Win High Scores." *New York Times,* April 8, 2003.

Pohl, Otto. "Improving the Way Humans Walk." *New York Times,* March 12, 2002.

Precision Striking. "Boxer Uppercut Tips: 5 Common Errors, Part 1 of 3." Video. October 11, 2017. https://youtu.be/GBRRy905Q2Q.

Precision Striking. "How to Wrap Your Hands for Boxing: Protect Your Hands for the Long Run." Video. February 3, 2018. https://youtu.be/mSxW47G0_NI.

Ramachandran, V. S. *The Tell-Tale Brain: A Neuroscientist's Quest for What Makes Us Human.* New York: W. W. Norton, 2011.

Robbins, Jeffrey, editor. *The Pleasure of Finding Things Out: The Best Short Works of Richard P. Feynman.* New York: Perseus, 1999.

Rodin, Auguste. *Pierre de Wiessant, nu monumental* (Pierre de Wiessant, monumental nude). Bronze sculpture. 1886. Brooklyn Museum, New York. https://tinyurl.com/uwvw94c.

Rodin, Auguste. *Le Penseur, nu monumental* (The Thinker, monumental nude). Bronze sculpture. 1902. New Yaohan, Macau.

Romanov, Nicholas. *Pose Method of Running.* Coral Gables, FL: Pose Method Publishing, 2004.

Sagan, Carl. *The Varieties of Scientific Experience: A Personal View of the Search for God.* Edited by Ann Druyan. New York: Penguin, 2006.

Schiffmann, Erich. *Yoga: The Spirit and Practice of Moving Into Stillness.* New York: Pocket, 1996.

Scott, Paul. "The Revolutionary New Science of Speed." *Men's Health,* January 31, 2011.

Sinnott, John. "Cracking Coaching's Final Frontier." BBC Sport, March 22, 2011. https://tinyurl.com/6hfxsxa.

Smith, Huston. *The Way Things Are: Conversations with Huston Smith on the Spiritual Life.* Edited by Philip Cousineau. Berkeley, CA: University of California Press, 2003.

Smith, Robert W. *Martial Musings: A Portrayal of the Martial Arts in the 20th Century.* Erie, PA: Via Media, 1999.

Snowden, Edward. *Permanent Record.* New York: Henry Holt & Co., 2019.

Waitzkin, Josh. *The Art of Learning: A Journey in the Pursuit of Excellence.* New York: Free Press, 2007.

Watts, Alan. *The Culture of Counter Culture: The Edited Transcripts.* Boston: Tuttle, 1998.

Watts, Alan. "A Cure for Education." *Talking Zen.* Excerpted in *Mountains Are Mountains and Rivers Are Rivers: Applying Eastern Teachings to Everyday Life.* Edited by Ilana Rabinowitz. New York: Hyperion, 1999.

Weinzweig, Ari. *Zingerman's Guide to Good Eating.* New York: Houghton Mifflin, 2003.

Willis, Adam. "Making the Perfect Sprinter More Perfect: How Usain Bolt Could Have Run Even Faster." *Slate*, August 5, 2017.

Wingfield, Adia Harvey, "How 'Service With a Smile' Takes a Toll on Women." *The Atlantic*, January 26, 2016.

Yu, Edward. *The Mass Psychology of Fittism: Fitness, Evolution, and the First Two Laws of Thermodynamics.* Undocumented Worker Press, 2015.

Index

About the Author

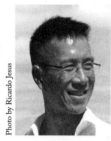

EDWARD YU is a former triathlete, current martial arts enthusiast, and perennial student of Masters Li Xueyi and Ge Guoliang in the art of Bagua, a.k.a. Baguazhang. Along with studying Bagua and Taichi, he has sampled enough boxing, kickboxing, and judo to know that sometimes it's better to run for your life.

The impetus for *Slowing Down to Run Faster* came years after Yu quit running and discovered that conventional approaches to training are not always effective in turning people into better athletes (even if they are often effective in making them discouraged and neurotic).

In his free time, Yu likes to roll on the floor, walk in circles, and stare into space.

ALSO BY EDWARD YU

The Mass Psychology of Fittism: Fitness Evolution and the First Two Laws of Thermodynamics

About North Atlantic Books

North Atlantic Books (NAB) is an independent, nonprofit publisher committed to a bold exploration of the relationships between mind, body, spirit, and nature. Founded in 1974, NAB aims to nurture a holistic view of the arts, sciences, humanities, and healing. To make a donation or to learn more about our books, authors, events, and newsletter, please visit www.northatlanticbooks.com.

North Atlantic Books is the publishing arm of the Society for the Study of Native Arts and Sciences, a 501(c)(3) nonprofit educational organization that promotes cross-cultural perspectives linking scientific, social, and artistic fields. To learn how you can support us, please visit our website.